Guiding the Young Athlete

Guiding the Young Athlete

All you need to know

David Jenkins and Peter Reaburn

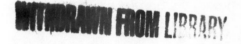
ALLEN & UNWIN

Copyright © David Jenkins and Peter Reaburn 2000

First published in 2000 by
Allen & Unwin
9 Atchison Street
St Leonards NSW 1590
Australia
Phone: (61 2) 8425 0100
Fax: (61 2) 9906 2218
E-mail: frontdesk@allen-unwin.com.au
Web: http://www.allen-unwin.com.au

National Library of Australia
Cataloguing-in-Publication entry:

Jenkins, David.
  Guiding the young athlete: all you need to know.
  Bibliography.
  ISBN 1 86508 218 X.

  1. Physical education and training. 2. Children— Physiology.
  3. Exercise for children. 4. Physical fitness for children.
  I. Reaburn, Peter. II. Title.

613.7042

Set in 11.5/15pt Garamond by DOCUPRO, Sydney
Printed and bound by Griffin Press Pty Ltd, Adelaide, SA

10 9 8 7 6 5 4 3 2 1

This book is dedicated to the memory of Dr John Leigh McNee, who passed away unexpectedly on 3 February 1999, aged 57.

Contents

Acknowledgments

The editors gratefully acknowledge the invaluable assistance of Judith Jenkins, who proofread the original manuscript; and Debbie Noon, who produced most of the figures.

David Jenkins, PhD, is a Senior Lecturer in Exercise Physiology at the University of Queensland. He was the senior scientific consultant to the Australian Rugby Football Union (ARFU) and the Australian Institute of Sport (Rugby) between 1988 and 1996. He is married with two very active young children.

Peter Reaburn, PhD, is a Senior Lecturer in Exercise Physiology within the School of Health and Human Performance at Central Queensland University in Rockhampton, Queensland. He is a member of the National Coaching Panel, AUSSI Masters swimming and was twice a finalist for the Queensland Sports Federation's Patron's award for Service to Sport. He is a high-performance masters triathlete with an active interest in surfboarding and endurance sports. He is married with two children and enjoys watching elite sports on television, reading Gerald Seymour novels and spending time with his family.

In the field of sports medicine, **Dr John McNee** will be remembered for his enormous commitment to the education of parents and coaches in the area of Children in Sport. He was a dynamic presenter who passionately defended the interests of youngsters. He was also extensively involved with Queensland Athletics and the Brisbane Strikers until his unexpected death on 3 February, 1999.

Preface

The purpose of this book is to provide information and advice to teachers, coaches and parents who wish to improve the fitness and health of young children and adolescents.

Scientists have long been aware of significant physiological differences between adults and children, yet most practical advice relating to fitness for children has been incomplete. In this book, we attempt to explain differences in the potential for exercise between children and adults and advice is offered on how children can exercise safely and effectively.

The book is organised into seven chapters. Chapter 1 compares key anatomical and physiological differences between girls and boys and between adults and children. These differences are important for understanding that activities and exercises performed by adults can be quite often dangerous for children. For example, performing low-intensity exercise in the heat carries a much greater risk of injury for children than it does for adults. This has clear implications for the timing of events for children, the frequency of rest breaks, availability of drinks and so on.

The main message carried by Chapter 2 is that exercise and sport can help give all children, irrespective of their health, some degree of functional and psychological independence. Improvements in general fitness, heart, lung and muscle function coupled with social and psychological development all contribute to a more complete development of the child. Chapter 2 also explains how children with the more common chronic health problems can make the most of the opportunities offered by exercise and sport.

Chapter 3 reviews common injuries which children unfortunately sometimes suffer in the course of normal sporting activities. While this chapter contains some material that is technical and is presented from a medical perspective, we feel that if the injuries and their treatments were described in any less detail, valuable information would be lost. It is not our intention that this chapter turns children away from exercise and sport. Rather, we hope that the explanations and advice we have included may help in promoting a rapid recovery to full health should a child become injured.

We review the methods for improving speed, endurance and flexibility in Chapter 4. These components of fitness, coupled with strength development (Chapter 5), are potential areas where children may be expected, unreasonably and often with a considerable degree of risk, to follow similar training practices to adults. By using and applying some of the material covered in Chapter 1, we explain what to do and what not to do when speed, endurance, flexibility and strength are developed with children. Children have a smaller capacity for muscle growth, their bones are immature and they have a lower capacity for the delivery and use of oxygen: these and other key physio-logical and anatomical differences all contribute to how we must view training with children differently to how we approach training with adults. In Chapters 4 and 5, there-fore, we explain what children can reasonably be expected to do and what they can realistically achieve. We also highlight the types of exercise which children must avoid.

In Chapter 6 we discuss techniques for enhancing recovery from training and competition. Recovery is one of the most important components of a training schedule. Children, by virtue of their enthusiasm, often become involved in a number of different activities. As well as being involved in several different sports, many children also engage in extracurricular activities such as music and drama lessons on top of their normal school requirements. Chap-ter 6 explains sensible techniques which can be used to prevent chronic tiredness and injury resulting from excessive activity.

Chapter 7 covers nutrition and exercise for children. We review a number of nutritional issues which are unique to childhood and adolescence and which impact upon the child's health as much as on his or her exercise capacity. This chapter also highlights specific nutritional problems and provides direction on how these can be avoided and/or resolved.

We hope the reader, be they a coach, parent or sports administrator, is enriched by the contents of this book. We also hope that the reader becomes acutely aware that *children are not little adults* and therefore need to be conditioned for sport differently than adults.

David Jenkins and Peter Reaburn

Changes to the body during childhood

David Jenkins and Peter Reaburn

This chapter looks at the main differences in anatomy and physiology between adults and children. It also discusses growth rates, or maturation and examines problems when children exercise in hot or cold conditions.

The human body undergoes an incredible series of changes during the lifespan. From the moment a child learns to move, his or her ability to control and refine their movements rapidly improves. Children demonstrate a remarkable ability to mimic actions and, while this is an essential part of learning, some exercises easily performed by adults should be avoided by or modified for children. This chapter will explain the more important anatomical and physiological differences between children and adults which impact upon how exercise should be prescribed to children. As we wrote in the Preface, children are not miniature adults. Due to differences in strength, maturity of bone, delivery and use of oxygen, the capacity to sweat and surface area/weight ratios, children and adults respond differently to exercise. This chapter will address those aspects which we feel explain why exercise training for children must differ, in most instances, from the schedules and routines used by adults.

COMPARISONS BETWEEN GIRLS AND BOYS

Height and weight

We can see from Figure 1 that boys and girls have similar increases in height up to 13 years of age; however, at 13, girls' height tends to plateau while boys' height continues to increase for a further two years. Changes in weight follow a similar pattern to those for height (Figure 2); increases

Figure 1 Average height of boys and girls between the ages of six and 18 years

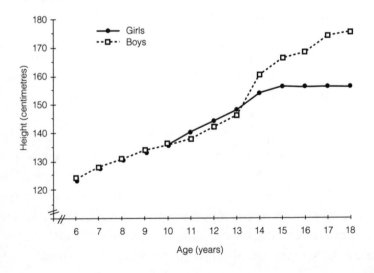

Figure 2 Average weight of boys and girls between the ages of six and 18 years

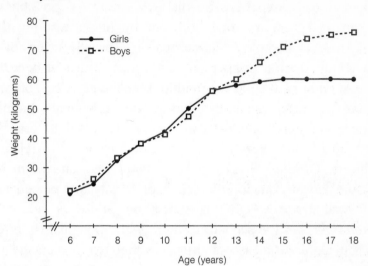

in weight are similar for boys and girls up to 14 years of age. Girls' weight then plateaus, while boys continue to gain weight until the age of 18. These two figures show average, or mean, changes in height and weight; remember that individual children may show considerable variation compared to these group values.

Growth

Growth and development are strongly related to genetic make-up. However, factors such as nutrition, disease, socioeconomic status and physical activity will all determine whether a child's genetic potential is reached.

Body fat levels

The amount of body fat we carry is important for two reasons: it influences exercise capacity, and it affects our health. In other words, too much body fat tends to slow us down and can bring on several diseases (for example, heart disease, hypertension, diabetes, etc.). It is possible to estimate a person's total body fat by first measuring the thickness of skinfold fat at various sites (usually seven) over the body. Special callipers are used to measure fat beneath the surface of the skin to within 1 millimetre. One of two things is then generally done. The individual skinfold numbers (in millimetres) can simply be added to provide a 'sum of skinfolds', which provides a measure of relative fatness. Or the values can be entered into one of many mathematical equations which express fat as a percentage of total body weight. The first procedure is normally preferred over the second, as there is the potential for error when skinfold measures are converted to percentage of body fat.

Figure 3 shows that the sum of skinfolds for boys gradually increases up to age 11 and then plateaus. In contrast, girls gain fat up to 15 years of age. Girls have slightly greater skinfold totals than boys across the entire

Figure 3 Average sum of triceps and subscapular skinfold thicknesses of boys and girls between the ages of six and 18 years

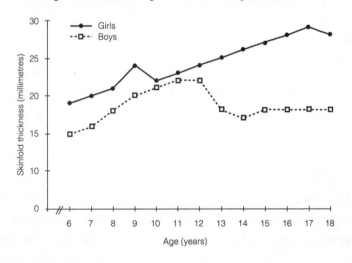

age range, though it is only after age 12 that this difference becomes pronounced.

Lohman (1986) has estimated that between the ages of six and 11 years, body fat in boys increases from 11 to 16 per cent, while for girls between the ages of six and 17 years, body fat increases from 14 to 27 per cent. Girls therefore carry more fat than boys into adulthood, and this difference is generally maintained during the lifespan.

Production of the hormone oestrogen increases in girls when they enter puberty, and this promotes relatively greater fat gains on their upper arms and the tops of their legs. Puberty for boys coincides with the release of the hormone testosterone, which promotes, among other things, growth of muscle.

Obesity

Research has shown that obese children eat no more than other children. However, it seems that there is a difference in activity levels between obese and non-obese children. Thus, energy intake would be similar, while energy expenditure would be lower for obese children. Increased body fat is related to the size and number of fat cells. In times of starvation or low energy (calorie) intake, the size of the fat cells decreases. Conversely, when we consume more energy than we use, the size of the fat cells increases. Thus, any imbalance between energy intake and energy expenditure will change the size of fat cells.

Interestingly, the *number* of fat cells increases rapidly during infancy and again during adolescence. Excessive intake of calories during these periods may result in a higher than desirable *increase* in the number of fat cells. The problem is that we are unable to *reduce* our fat cell number; once we have them, we are stuck with them. In other words, we will always then have a tendency to be overweight. So, by making sure that energy intake and expenditure are well balanced during childhood and adolescence, we can prevent too great an increase in the number of our fat cells.

Muscle strength

It is easier to estimate the amount of fat we carry than the amount of muscle we have. Strength tests have typically been used to gauge changes in muscle tissue as a result of growth and strength training; such tests have included the 'flexed arm hang', 'sit-ups' and 'hand-grip' strength. Even though both boys and girls show similar improvements in performance in these tests up to 12 years of age, boys consistently score 10 per cent higher than girls in hand-grip strength.

Sociological issues tend to complicate comparison of strength between boys and girls. In other words, when we compare strength between boys and girls, we must remember that boys generally participate in activities that require a fair degree of strength; usually to a greater extent than many girls do. To overcome this bias, throwing distance using the non-dominant hand is typically used to assess the relationship between gender and strength. For example, when pre-adolescent boys and girls of the same age throw a ball with their non-dominant hand, the distances reached are very similar. Predictably, boys throw further than girls with their dominant hand, and this has been attributed to differences in practice and greater involvement in activities that involve throwing. If it was simply a gender difference, then we would expect boys to throw further than girls with their non-dominant as well as their dominant hand. What is not as easily explained is why boys should score consistently higher in non-dominant hand-grip strength.

Bone density

The density of bone (or bone mineral density, BMD) increases steadily for both boys and girls from birth to puberty. During puberty, BMD rapidly increases (by up to 15 per cent) and, due to early maturation, girls experience their gain in bone mineralisation approximately three years before boys. While physical activity before the onset of puberty does not appear to significantly increase BMD, it has been estimated that activity *during* puberty could increase it by 10 per cent. That is, active children come through puberty with 10 per cent greater BMD than less active children. Two points are important here. First, research has shown that weight-bearing activities are particularly effective in increasing BMD. Second, adolescence must be the time for maximising gains in BMD so as to provide 'protection' against osteoporosis later in life. Up to 90 per cent of adult bone is deposited by the end of adolescence.

There are several factors which prevent youngsters achieving peak bone mass (that is, maximal gains in BMD). First, smoking impairs the release of oestrogen, which in turn reduces gains in bone, particularly with females. Second, excessive consumption of soft drinks will reduce the retention of calcium and the formation of new bone. The reason is that soft drinks have a high phosphorus content, and phosphorus reduces the concentrations of calcium in the blood, which in turn causes a release of calcium from bone (that is, bone loss). Third, girls who menstruate fewer than six times a year will run an increased risk of losing bone; this again is related to reduced levels of oestrogen. For a girl to return to regular menstruation, she may need to reduce her training load and increase her energy intake to gain body mass, including fat. (See Chapter 7 for advice on the nutritional requirements of young athletes.)

Loss of BMD is strongly related to eating disorders, which is not surprising given that nutrition plays such a central role in maximising growth. Factors that maintain and promote bone growth include adequate energy (that is, calorie intake), protein, vitamin D and calcium intake. Energy is required for the growth of all tissues, including bone. The bone matrix is made of protein, so the diet must meet the protein needs of the body. Vitamin D is necessary for the manufacture of bone and is gained from both sunlight and the diet; a number of foods, such as cereals and milk, are naturally fortified with vitamin D. Finally, calcium intake is particularly important during periods of growth, although the precise levels needed to maximise increases in BMD are not available.

Development of coordination and skill

A child's ability to develop skill is more closely related to biological age (that is, maturity) than to chronological age, and children of the same age will rarely share the same ability to learn and develop a particular skill. Sociocultural factors, which include past experiences, opportunities to practise, and so forth, will also strongly influence skill development.

When compared to adults, children have a poorer capacity to concentrate and to understand complex arrangements of movement. Practice will be a complete waste of time for children who are not capable of learning a new skill; instead, they are likely to become frustrated, and attempts to return to the task when they are older will be difficult. Early learning is largely experimental, and it is when a child wants to jump over something or throw a ball to hit a target that skill training in a related activity should be introduced.

Factors such as size, shape and body composition change up to and beyond adolescence. Moreover, these factors develop at different times, so it makes sense that there are 'critical' times during which certain skills can be learned and practised effectively. Thus, training must coincide with the appropriate physical and mental age for the child.

Changes in the ability of a child to balance are at least partially related to changes in his or her centre of gravity. As children age, the centre of gravity gets lower; at five years of age, the centre of gravity is near the belly button, while at age 13, it is horizontal to the top of the hip. Some researchers have suggested that this is why a younger child finds it more difficult to balance in an upright position than an older child, and this has been used to explain the relative ease with which certain skills that require balance are learned by older children.

As the child grows, skills will have to be modified to accommodate the changes in size and body composition. There is a reasonable case for not investing too much time in perfecting a particular skill too early, because it will always need to be relearned. It is better to promote enjoyment, rather than perfection of skill, during periods of rapid growth. Activities should include throwing, catching, jumping and running, and tasks that require balance.

The period between ages seven and 11 is good for skill development. Up to the age of nine, children execute movements with little thought of the outcome. However, beyond nine years of age, their attention is directed towards making skills more efficient and to achieving a given level of performance. At this age, children want to do well at sports even though their attention span is not particularly impressive. They tend not to appreciate long-term objectives or outcomes of a given activity. At around age 11, competition and team games become more important; children begin to learn about cooperation and the collective aims of the team, and to develop socialising skills.

It is generally agreed that up to adolescence, children should be given every opportunity to learn a wide variety of physical skills. This broad base allows different interests to be followed in the future, particularly when an earlier activity is no longer possible or attractive. Specialisation too early in childhood can limit later opportunities.

Coordination will continue during periods of rapid growth, even if it seems that children are becoming more clumsy and regressing. This is not the case; it is just that the *rate* of improvement during such periods may be slower than before.

There are no apparent differences in the rate of skill development between boys and girls. In other words, both are capable of learning a skill at the same speed. However, some skills (overarm throwing for boys and skipping for girls) have a heavy cultural bias, and so there will be differences in ability when certain skills are compared between boys and girls. Having said that, the interests of boys and girls are probably more similar between ten and 12 years than at any other age.

EXERCISE AND HEART AND LUNG FUNCTION

All structures and functioning of a child, including the lungs, heart and blood vessels, undergo many changes as they develop. The purpose of this section is to examine the changes that occur in the systems that deliver oxygen to the exercising muscles—the cardiovascular (heart–blood) and respiratory systems.

How the cardiovascular system works

The functioning of the cardiovascular system during exercise can be broken down into a number of separate yet related factors. These include:

- **Maximal oxygen consumption** is the maximal volume of oxygen that can be transported to, and consumed by, the working tissues. The more oxygen that can be transported to, and consumed by, the exercising muscles, the better for the young endurance athlete.
- **Cardiac output (CO)**, which is the volume of blood that is pumped by the heart each minute. CO depends on the heart rate per minute and on how much blood is pumped per beat of the heart—a concept called stroke volume. The more blood that can be pumped per minute, the more oxygen is available to be taken up by the muscles.
- **Arteriovenous oxygen difference** is simply the amount of oxygen extracted by the muscles from the available blood (cardiac output). As the name suggests, it is the difference in oxygen content of the blood between the arterial concentration of oxygen and the concentration of oxygen in the blood of the veins. The more oxygen a muscle can extract, the better for the young endurance athlete.
- **Blood pressure** is simply the pressure exerted by the blood on the blood vessels of the body. If blood pressure is too high, the heart has to work hard to overcome the pressure and, as such, the health of the heart is compromised.

We will now examine how each of these factors is affected by exercise and consider the changes that occur with a child's growth.

Responses to exercise

1 Maximal oxygen consumption, in terms of the number of litres of oxygen consumed per minute, increases with age up until approximately 20 years (Figure 4). After this age, it appears to decline at around 1 per cent per year in non-exercisers and by about 0.5 per cent per year in athletes.

Importantly, at around 12–15 years of age, boys appear to improve their aerobic capacity at a much faster rate than girls. Some researchers suggest that this may reflect the social phenomenon of boys being more physically active than girls at that age, but other differences also occur with boys. For example, heart size and blood oxygen-carrying capacity increase at a faster rate in boys than in girls.

Figure 4 Changes in aerobic capacity (litres per minute) in boys and girls between the ages of six and 18 years

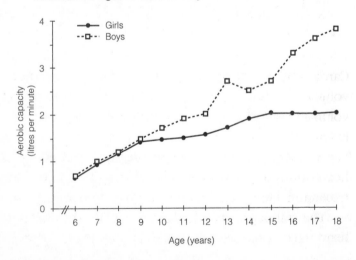

In sports science, we generally express maximal oxygen consumption relative to body weight. That is, instead of litres per minute, we use millilitres per kilogram per minute. Figure 5 suggests that the aerobic capacity of males (millilitres per kilogram per minute) remains fairly constant throughout growth, while in females it decreases significantly, particularly as girls naturally put on body fat (non-oxygen using) at around 12 years of age.

Figure 5 Changes in aerobic capacity (millilitres per kilogram per minute) in boys and girls between the ages of six and 18 years

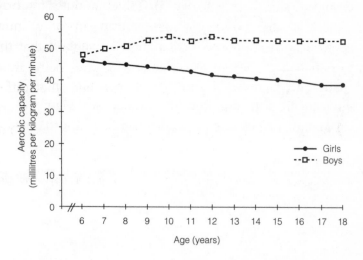

2 Cardiac output is the product of heart rate and stroke volume. A child's smaller heart size and smaller blood volume result in the stroke volume of a child being lower than that of an adult. However, a child's heart has the ability to pump more quickly than an adult's heart at any level of exercise. Children also have higher maximum heart rates than adults.

The standard way of estimating a person's maximum heart rate is to deduct their age from 220. However, this is a rough estimate only, and there can be an enormous range of 'normal'. In some sports such as swimming, coaches prescribe training intensity by specifying '20 below' or '40 below', say, which means 20 or 40 beats below maximum. It is doubtful whether the same coaches appreciate that this sort of prescription assumes they actually know the maximum heart rate of their athlete. Assuming the maximum heart rate is 220 minus age leads to large errors in prescribing training intensities. The best way of finding maximum heart rate is by doing a test of maximal heart rate by doing a small set of two- to three-minute intervals ('intervals' are bouts of high-intensity exercise interspersed with short recovery periods), increasing speed to exhaustion.

3 Heart rate increases linearly with increases in exercise intensity in both children and adults (see Figure 6).

Maximal heart rate appears to drop by approximately

Figure 6 Heart rate response to increased exercise intensity in children and adults

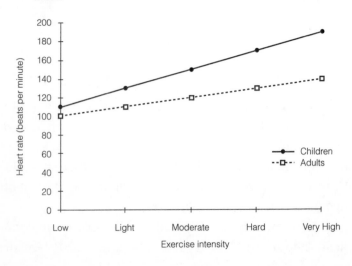

one beat per year as a child ages. This decline is independent of gender, fitness level or race.

There appears to be a gender difference in heart rate response to exercise. For example, girls of any age appear to have a higher heart rate than boys for the same speed of training. It has been suggested that this may be due to the fact that boys have:

• higher stroke volumes compared to girls, meaning that more blood is pumped per beat;
• greater nervous system stimulation of the heart;
• after 12–15 years of age, a higher haemoglobin (oxygen-carrying protein) concentration in the blood; and
• after 12–15 years of age, a higher muscle mass that can take up more oxygen.

It has also been suggested that boys' heart rates recover more quickly than girls' heart rates after exercise.

4 Stroke volume increases as exercise intensity increases in both adults and children (Figure 7). This increase, at

Figure 7 Stroke volume response to increased exercise intensity in children and adults

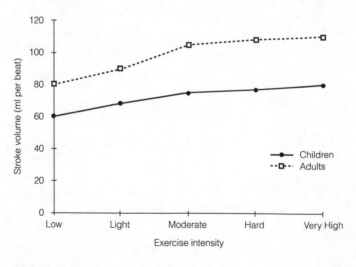

least in elite athletes, appears to continue up until maximal exercise, with a suggestion that in non-elite athletes, stroke volume may plateau at moderate exercise intensities.

5 Arteriovenous oxygen difference is significantly higher in children compared to adults (Figure 8). This means that children can extract more oxygen from the blood than adults. It also means they are better at getting oxygen into their muscles more quickly than adults, and they can recover from efforts during training more quickly. Finally, it suggests that children will not produce as much lactic acid as adults at the start of hard exercise.

6 Blood pressure while at rest and during exercise is lower in children than in adults. This is partially due to the fact that the blood vessel walls of children are more elastic than those of adults, whose artery walls tend to harden with age. However, as the child develops to

Figure 8 Arteriovenous oxygen difference response to increased exercise intensity in children and adults

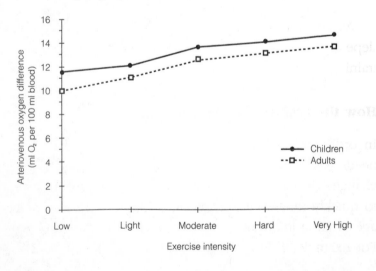

adulthood, the blood pressure values increase. Blood pressure depends greatly on body size, so we would expect larger children to have higher blood pressure at rest and during exercise than smaller children of the same age.

Cardiovascular adaptations to training in children

The response of children to endurance training or physical training of long duration is similar to that of adults. The following changes have been observed in studies that have trained children over time:

- increased blood volume (thus increasing oxygen-carrying capacity);
- increasing total haemoglobin (thus increasing oxygen-carrying capacity);
- increased stroke volume (at least in pubertal children);
- lower resting heart rates;
- faster heart rate recovery;
- increased heart size independent of normal growth; and
- increased maximal oxygen consumption.

As in adults, these changes will differ in children, depending on the intensity, duration and frequency of training, as well as genetic factors.

How the respiratory system works

In order for oxygen to be taken up by the blood, it first needs to be taken into the lungs via breathing. Lung function changes as children age, with lung capacity and the ability to quickly inhale and exhale all increasing with advancing age until adulthood, after which it gradually decreases. For example, a five-year-old boy has the ability to take in about 40 litres of air per minute, and this increases to about 120 litres per minute at 25 years of age.

Girls follow the same general pattern as boys, but their values, particularly after puberty, are lower due to their smaller body size and height.

THE EFFECTS ON CHILDREN OF EXERCISING IN EXTREME TEMPERATURES

Children, like adults, exercise during the summer months. However, unlike adults, children do not appear to cope as well as adults with exercise in hot and humid climates. This relative intolerance to heat is due to a number of physiological differences between children and adults. Some of these differences that are relevant to exercising in hot or cold temperatures include children having:

- a reduced ability to sweat;
- a greater body surface area-to-weight ratio, meaning they have more skin surface area to gain or lose heat;
- a lower sweat rate;
- the ability to start sweating at a higher temperature;
- a reduced thirst mechanism; and
- the ability to acclimatise more slowly.

As a result of these differences, children react to exercising in hot or cold air or water completely differently to adults. For example, in a cool environment, their large body surface area-to-weight ratio means they will lose heat faster than most adults. This can be an advantage in cool conditions (say 20–25 degrees Celsius), but if the temperature is cold, they can lose a lot of heat and be at risk of cold injuries (see below).

The high surface area-to-weight ratio is also a disadvantage when exercising in the heat. Once the air or water temperature gets above skin temperature (about 32–33 degrees Celsius), children gain heat from the environment. Their reduced ability to sweat, combined with their starting to sweat at a higher temperature than adults, places them at an increased risk of heat injury (see below for symptoms).

In summary, it appears that children may be more at risk of heat and cold injuries than adults. However, the number of scientific studies examining the response of children to exercise in the heat and the cold are limited, and the reported cases of heat injury are small given the number of participants in junior sport. A conservative approach is recommended when advising children about safe exercise habits in temperature extremes.

Exercising in hot and/or humid conditions

Children exercising in hot and/or humid conditions are more at risk of heat injury than are adults, and precautions are obviously recommended. This is particularly the case in children with heavy or solid builds who have a large muscle mass that generates a lot of heat. Children with high levels of body fat not only have the problem of having extra insulation from the fat, but are generally less conditioned than leaner children. Certain illnesses such as cystic fibrosis, anorexia nervosa (slimming disease), diabetes and congenital heart disease also make children more susceptible to heat illness when exercising in the heat. Children with these illnesses need to be monitored particularly carefully.

Heat illness can be very serious and may lead to medical intervention. It is therefore essential that coaches, sports administrators and parents are aware of the early warning signs of heat illness in children.

Early warning signs of heat illness in children

- tiredness;
- weakness;
- headache;
- muscle or stomach cramping;
- nausea;
- bright red skin;
- excessive sweating; and
- possible fainting.

If any of the indicators of heat illness appear, then the following actions are recommended:

1 Remove the child from the field, court or event.
2 Lay them down in a cool, well-ventilated place.
3 Expose their skin by removing clothing.
4 Give them cool water.
5 Place wet towels over their exposed skin.
6 Sponge them with cool water.

Strategies for preventing heat illness
Prevention is better then cure. Sports Medicine Australia recently produced an excellent publication called *Safety Guidelines for Children in Sport and Recreation*. This publication recommends the following guidelines when children are exercising in the heat:

- Watch them closely for signs of heat illness.
- Use non-oil-based sunscreens (available from chemists), as the oil-based ones can block the sweat pores. The SPF (Sun Protection Factor) should exceed 15.
- Wear hats where appropriate.

- Wear light-coloured, loose-fitting, natural fibre (cotton or wool) or specially designed fabrics (CoolMax™ or Dri-Fit™), not nylons or rayons which hold heat.
- Ensure that children drink fluids before, during and after training or competing to prevent dehydration.

Other strategies for prevention of heat illness include acclimatisation, monitoring weight loss and fluid replacement.

Acclimatisation: By exercising regularly (three to six times a week) in the heat for short periods, starting at a slow pace then gradually increasing exercise intensity and duration, the body will acclimatise by increasing its sweat rate and body water content. This process takes longer in children (14 days) than adults (seven to ten days).

Monitoring weight loss: One kilogram of body weight lost equals approximately one litre of fluid lost. The aim should be to maintain body weight as close to normal as possible by fluid replacement.

Fluid replacement: Children's thirst mechanism is not as well developed as that of adults. They also appear to have a lower tolerance for fluid in the stomach than do adults, making fluid replacement even more difficult. Sports Medicine Australia thus recommends the fluid intake schedule shown in Table 1 for children involved with events lasting less than one hour.

Table 1 Suggested fluid intake guidelines before, during and after sport

	Average 10-year-old	Average 15-year-old
Before event (45 mins)	150–200 ml water	300–400 ml water
During event	75–100 ml water every 20 minutes	150–200 ml water every 20 minutes
After event	Drink water until urine is clear	Drink water until urine is clear

Sports drinks such as Gatorade™ or Powerade™ may also be used, since they are more palatable and may encourage fluid intake in children.

The role of officials

On particularly hot and/or humid days, sports administrators or event organisers can also help to prevent heat illness in children by:

1 Educating parents, coaches and medical personnel as to the signs of heat illness and the prevention/treatment strategies.

2 Ensuring that the medical coverage group meets with coaches and officials to discuss the following:

- additional water breaks;
- more frequent breaks or time-outs;
- turning the halves into quarters;
- changing the starting time to a cooler time of the day; and
- availability of shaded areas in well-ventilated positions.

3 Ensuring that the medical coverage team have the following on hand:

- intravenous solutions;
- cooling aids, such as ice packs, fans or kiddies' pools;
- cool water;
- shaded rest areas; and
- medical transportation and access.

4 Preventing or minimising the wearing of taping, padding, sweatbands, bandanas, gloves, etc., that help to store heat.

In conclusion, heat illness in children is avoidable. Thoughtful prevention and observation strategies are the responsibility of the parent, coach and sports administrator. Adherence to the strategies outlined above will go a long way towards ensuring that children are able to safely play, train or compete in hot conditions.

Exercising in cold conditions

Children are also more susceptible than adults to illness in cold climates. This applies most importantly to lean or thin children whose high body surface area-to-weight ratio allows them to lose heat quickly in cold air or water. Research has also shown that children have a less developed perception of when they are cold and may therefore keep playing or stay in the water longer than they should.

When anyone, particularly children, exercises in the cold air or water, a number of factors may predispose them to cold injury. These factors include:

- air or water temperature;
- wind velocity—windchill is a major risk, particularly when wet;
- lack of protective clothing;
- wet body or clothing;
- prolonged exposure;
- fatigue;
- dehydration;
- lack of carbohydrate;
- contact with cold surfaces, such as water or ice; and
- low intensity of exercise.

The astute coach or parent must be aware, as with heat injuries, that if these risk factors are present, signs or symptoms suggesting cold injury may appear.

Early warning signs of cold illness in children

- weak pulse;
- slurred speech;
- cold skin temperatures;
- blueness of the lips;
- irrational thinking; and
- decreased performance.

Treatment of mild hypothermia is via the following means:

- Gradual warming by blankets or a warm bath.
- Removal from the wind.
- Removal of wet clothing and replacing with warm, dry clothing.
- Gradual intake of warm fluids.

Application of external heat via a heater, enforced exercise, rubbing of the skin or alcohol intake can be dangerous, due to these treatments possibly causing further heat loss from the skin.

Strategies for preventing cold illness
Sports Medicine Australia's *Safety Guidelines for Children in Sport and Recreation* make the following recommendations when exercising in wet or cold conditions:

1 Avoid standing exposed for long periods.
2 Change wet clothing as soon as practicable.
3 Wear appropriate clothing:
   - Dress in layers to trap heat between them.
   - Add or remove layers as the exercise intensity or temperature conditions demand.

- Wear or remove a waterproof jacket and/or hood as demanded by the conditions.
- Wear clothes with clips, zips or drawstrings (at the waist, arm, neck, etc.) so that they can be loosened or tightened as necessary.
- Wear hats and gloves to reduce heat loss.

In conclusion, while not as common as heat injury, cold injuries in children can occur given that they are at a greater risk than adults. Again, prevention is the key, through staying dry and by wearing appropriate clothing. However, if the signs of cold injury appear, the astute coach or parent should remove the child from the playing field, dry them in a windless area, cover them with warm blankets or clothing, and ensure that they take in warm fluids.

SUMMARY

✓ Girls and boys have similar increases in height and weight up to around the age of 13. Thereafter, differences in height, weight, fat and muscle mass are evident between males and females.

✓ Fat cells increase in number in early infancy and again in adolescence. It is possible that poor nutrition and inactivity, particularly in the early teenage years, may contribute to obesity later in life.

✓ It is essential that children and teenagers maximise the amount of calcium stored in their bones. Both exercise and a high intake of calcium in the diet help to achieve a high bone mineral density. Smoking and too many soft drinks decrease the amount of calcium stored in bone.

✓ Up to adolescence, children should be given every opportunity to learn a wide variety of physical skills. Specialisation too early can limit later opportunities.

✓ Exercise in children produces a linear increase in aerobic capacity, cardiac output, heart rate and arteriovenous oxygen difference. It appears that children have a significantly lower stroke volume than do adults, due to their smaller heart and body size. However, they are capable of significantly higher maximal heart rates than adults and have a much greater arteriovenous oxygen difference than adults. This suggests that they are highly aerobic, which is reflected in their ability to both adjust to exercise quickly and recover more quickly between efforts than adults.

✓ Children appear to adapt to physical training in the same way as adults do. They demonstrate positive changes in heart size and function, as well as increases in factors that affect the blood's oxygen-carrying capacity.

✓ Children exercising in hot and/or humid conditions are more at risk of heat injury than adults; children are generally less efficient and sweat less.

✓ Children are also more susceptible than adults to illness in cold climates. They have high body surface area-to-weight ratios which lead to more rapid heat loss in cold air or water.

2

Chronic health disorders and exercise

Dr John McNee

This chapter looks at particular health problems and explains how children with health disorders can exercise safely.

INTRODUCTION

Up to 10 per cent of children have some long-term physical or psychological health problem. In this chapter we will look at only the following, more common, physical disorders:

- asthma
- heart disease
- cystic fibrosis
- epilepsy
- diabetes

- arthritis
- haemophilia

Information on the effects of exercise on other health problems is available through more specific sources (such as sporting organisations for the hearing impaired, the visually impaired and the intellectually impaired).

There is an understandable tendency among parents, teachers, health practitioners and coaches to be overprotective of children with a chronic illness or physical disability. Even if the child does not have a life-threatening disorder, we often want to prevent further suffering and pain—especially since sport and exercise may be associated with injury. However, exercise is essential for growth and development, for general fitness, for good heart and lung function, for muscle growth and strength, and for social and psychological development. Team or group activities also allow a child to develop social and organisational skills. Furthermore, involvement in sport allows a child to gain self-esteem and independence. In other words, exercise and sport can help a child with chronic health problems to grow into an independent adult within the limits of their illness or disability.

ASTHMA

Asthma is the most common chronic respiratory disease among children younger than 19 years of age and, for unknown reasons, the incidence of asthma is slowly increasing. It is believed that asthma has a genetic background, and at some stage during life something triggers the development of the disease. The most common triggers are viral infections, but other stimuli such as allergy reactions to inhaled or ingested substances may also be involved.

Asthma is not just one disease but a spectrum of clinical states with a wide variety of symptoms, signs and outcomes. The National Heart and Lung Institute of America defines asthma as a lung disease characterised by:

- airway obstruction;
- complete or partial reversibility of the airway obstruction;
- airway inflammation; and
- increased airway responsiveness to a variety of stimuli (or triggers).

Most children with asthma have some degree of exercise-induced asthma (EIA, or bronchospasm). This means that exercise may act as a trigger to produce the bronchospasm. Some asthmatics only experience airway obstruction when they exercise, while others experience obstruction at rest as well.

The effects of exercise

Exercise-induced asthma is triggered by an increased rate of breathing, a drop in air temperature, evaporation of fluid from cells in the breathing tubes and, finally, contraction of the airways. This then causes respiratory distress, wheezing or coughing, or all of these. Whatever the symptoms, the ability to continue to exercise is reduced.

In competitive sports, medications for the management of asthma can be used as inhaled drugs, but oral or intravenous drugs are not permitted. The relevant sporting association must be notified if an athlete who competes at national or international level uses a bronchodilator.

Provided the asthma is well controlled, research has shown that endurance training can produce the same improvements in heart and lung function in well-controlled asthmatic children as in non-asthmatic children. Indeed, up to 10 per cent of Olympic-level athletes have asthma or exercise-induced asthma.

The potential benefits of exercise in children with asthma include improved self-esteem, improved cardiopulmonary fitness, decreased severity and frequency of asthma attacks, and a decrease in medication use. In some asthmatic children, when they first start an activity program they may develop a mild asthma attack; however, if they continue with the activity, the asthma will disappear and they will be able to maintain exercise at a much higher level. This is known as the refractory period and is used by many asthmatic athletes. These athletes develop a mild asthma attack during the warm-up prior to an activity before entering the refractory period (which coincides with the activity itself). Exercise can then be continued for two to three hours without medication or distress. This refractory period will only occur if the asthma is well controlled and is only experienced by 40–50 per cent of asthmatics.

Recommendations and precautions

Appropriate medications should be used to control asthma. Exercise-induced asthma may require specific medication (for example, Intal, Ventolin, Serevent or Bricanyl) 30–40 minutes prior to exercise. The athlete will not require any further medication for at least three to four hours.

Asthmatics should avoid using medication (for example, Ventolin or Bricanyl) *during* the activity; children should be strongly urged not to carry asthma puffers when doing their activity.

Climatic conditions influence asthma. For example, very cold and very dry air can bring on an attack. Training should therefore be avoided at times when the air is dry and cold. Air pollution (such as pollen) can also bring on an asthma attack; training during certain times in the spring and summer may therefore need to be avoided, or at least reduced.

Indoor activities in well-ventilated or air-conditioned environments are generally well tolerated. However, indoor swimming in pools with a high chlorine content may cause problems for some children; chlorine in outdoor pools is less problematic, but some children may be affected. Swimming in a warm, humid environment is a suitable activity for most asthmatics; however, it is a myth that swimming 'cures' asthma.

In general, asthmatics can participate in most physical activities and sports. However, some sports that require high-intensity exercise and rapid breathing over an extended period (for example, cross-country running or road cycling) or which involve exercise in cool, dry air (such as ice sports or winter endurance running) can produce asthma. Aerobic (endurance) exercise should not cause significant problems provided the activity is not maintained for long periods of time. Activities that improve breathing techniques and control are recommended for asthmatics.

HEART DISORDERS

Most children and young adults who have a chronic cardiac disorder have a congenital structural defect. Others will have acquired the disorder during childhood as a result of bacteria and viruses, drugs and drug abuse, chemicals and, rarely, coronary artery disease.

Most children who have chronic heart disorders have very low exercise tolerance and poor fitness levels on testing. Although part of this may be directly related to the cardiac pathology, under-activity caused by over-protection from parents, health personnel and educators is the main reason for the children's poor fitness.

Specific disorders

Marfan's syndrome

Marfan's syndrome is a hereditary disorder which affects the bones, joints, eyes, heart and blood vessels. Those who are most affected are usually tall, and therefore are likely to participate in those sports where height is an advantage (for example, basketball, volleyball, high jump, etc.). As there are wide variations in the clinical features of Marfan's syndrome, some children and adolescents may show no other obvious signs of the disorder except tallness. Children who are particularly tall should therefore be screened by a sports physician. Identification of the disorder is important, given the higher than normal risk of cardiac problems (including sudden death). Children who are diagnosed with Marfan's syndrome should be encouraged to participate in suitable activities such as recreational swimming, cycling, golf or archery.

Hypertrophic cardiomyopathy

Hypertrophic cardiomyopathy is a disease of the heart muscle. It is thought to be strongly determined by genetics. The problem is related to a thickening of the muscle that makes up the left ventricle (pumping chamber), which in turn leads to inadequate filling and reduced pumping of the blood around the body. Hypertrophic cardiomyopathy is a condition that is associated with sudden death.

Recommendations as to the level of suitable activity will depend on the clinical symptoms, signs and investigations.

However, low-intensity, non-competitive activities such as walking, recreational swimming and golf are allowable for most individuals, except those with severe disease.

Sudden death

The four most common causes of sudden death are:

- hypertrophic cardiomyopathy;
- coronary artery anomalous anatomy;
- aortic dissection (Marfan's syndrome); and
- premature atherosclerosis (coronary artery disease).

These conditions are not common, and in many situations are not known to be present, and few, if any, symptoms are apparent prior to death.

It is important to realise that the most common cardiac conditions usually are not responsible for sudden death in young athletes.

The effects of exercise

Suitable exercise programs have been shown to improve heart function and blood supply to the muscles of most children with congenital heart disease. Such improvements in response to carefully constructed training programs allow children with heart problems to participate in a wide variety of physical activities and sports before they reach a point where the underlying cardiac condition limits their level of activity.

Recommendations and precautions

As is the case with adults, good exercise rehabilitation is important after any surgical procedures.

Before a child with heart disease begins an exercise

program, it is necessary to consult with the child's doctors to gain advice on the level of activity. Most congenital heart conditions have now been well researched, and information is available as to what is appropriate.

As some congenital defects do tend to improve with growth and development, it is important to increase the level of activity as the condition improves.

Some cardiac disorders will limit the child to a low level of activity, but it is important to encourage the child to reach that level.

CYSTIC FIBROSIS

Cystic fibrosis is the most common genetically inherited disease leading to early death in our population; it occurs in approximately 1 in 2500 live births. The problem relates to transport of water across compartments in the body, which leads to dehydration. This affects the functions of the lungs, the pancreas, the intestinal mucosal cells (by increasing the viscosity of the secretions of these cells) and the sweat glands (by causing them to secrete abnormally high levels of salt and water). In addition, intestinal problems lead to poor absorption of nutrients.

Disease of the breathing airways may cause nasal polyps, sinusitis, airway obstructions and lung infections, each contributing to a progressive loss of lung function.

Reduced exercise capacity with cystic fibrosis can therefore be attributed to:

- low levels of oxygen in the blood;
- increasing cough;
- shortness of breath; and
- salt and fluid loss.

The effects of exercise

Many of the potential problems associated with cystic fibrosis can be anticipated and largely prevented. For example, bronchodilators (puffers) can be used before exercise to ensure that exercise levels are maintained at a point where sufficient oxygen reaches the muscles. In addition, children with cystic fibrosis need to drink fluids with electrolytes (such as sports drinks) frequently.

Exercise in children with cystic fibrosis improves exercise tolerance and lung function, reduces breathlessness, can help improve sputum clearance and can improve the quality of life.

Recommendations and precautions

With the exception of diving, children with cystic fibrosis do not have to avoid any particular type of exercise. However, some activities may need to be modified, depending on the state of the disease at any given time. Collision sports need not be avoided for children where the disease is well controlled. It is important that supervisors in the sport allow children with cystic fibrosis to use their medications when necessary, to have breaks as they require and to replace their fluids frequently during exercise.

EPILEPSY

There are many forms of epilepsy in childhood and adolescence. While some are relatively minor, others can result in seizures (convulsions). All forms of epilepsy are due to abnormal electrical activity in the brain. Most childhood epilepsies respond very well to anti-epileptic medication, and most children do not have brain damage or an intellectual disability. Some epilepsies are not life-long and the disorder may improve or disappear during puberty.

The incidence of sudden unexplained death in epileptics is found usually in adults with a long history of convulsive disorders and poor compliance with anti-epileptic medication. It is not a common problem in children and adolescents. Drowning rates have been reported as being relatively high in epileptics, either bathtub drownings or lone swimming. However, other reports have shown little or no increase in drownings among epileptics as a result of a seizure.

The effects of exercise

Many anecdotal accounts and some studies suggest that exercise improves the control of epilepsy and reduces the number of seizures. However, this is not supported by the scientific evidence.

What is known is that seizure-related injuries are not increased in epileptics who participate in sport. Most authorities now accept that if the seizures are well controlled (for example, no seizure in the last 12 months), a child should be permitted to participate in all sporting activities. Obviously, if the seizures are more frequent and the problem is not well controlled, there will need to be certain restrictions on exercise. The following questions can be helpful in considering restrictions:

- Is there potential for injury to the child, to team-mates or to spectators if a convulsion occurs?
- Are there significant side-effects to the medication, particularly when fine motor skills and coordination are required?
- Does the child have any particular physical skills, motivations or disabilities?

It should be remembered that in our culture, epileptics experience a significant bias against them. Because of this, the epileptic child should be encouraged to participate in any type of activity that will enhance his or her self-esteem and self-worth.

Recommendations and precautions

Before beginning an exercise program, the child's parents, teachers or coach should discuss the extent of the child's condition with a sports physician or neurologist. The carers should also know first-aid management of an epileptic seizure.

The child must be prepared to diligently observe the medication regime and not miss taking tablets.

It is important that adolescent epileptics do not take alcohol, or use recreational drugs or anabolic steroids, as these will interfere with the anti-epileptic medication and may increase the number of seizures.

DIABETES MELLITUS

Diabetes is a disorder characterised by the body's inability to regulate blood glucose levels. The hormone insulin may be absent or have a decreased action, and the use of carbohydrate, fat and protein by the body is usually disturbed. If diabetes is not well controlled, serious long-term health complications will result.

There are two types of diabetes:

- insulin-dependent diabetes mellitus (IDDM); and
- non-insulin-dependent diabetes mellitus (NIDDM).

IDDM is the most common form in children. Much work is being done to establish the cause of this condition and to improve the future management of it. Major improvements in our understanding of the condition are likely to occur over the next five to ten years.

The effects of exercise

It is known that exercise makes the body more sensitive to injected insulin and may allow a lower amount of insulin to be used to maintain optimum control of blood glucose. However, exercise itself may cause hypoglycaemia (low blood glucose) or hyperglycaemia (high blood glucose) and make it difficult to maintain normal glucose levels. Nonetheless, given the availability of multiple-dose insulins, insulin pump therapy and self-monitoring of blood glucose levels, it is possible for diabetic children to have good control over their blood glucose levels, and thus be able to participate at any level of sporting activity.

It is well accepted that any form of exercise or sporting activity is suitable for diabetics, provided the condition is well controlled. In addition, regular exercise will assist in the control or prevention of obesity and coronary artery disease, which must be avoided by diabetics.

Recommendations and precautions

Children with IDDM need to pay particular attention to their pre-exercise meal and carbohydrate feeding during exercise. Both will influence blood glucose levels. They may also need to decrease their pre-exercise insulin dose (because exercise enhances the action of insulin). Glucose levels will need to be monitored during exercise to determine the individual response to exercise.

Glucose levels will need to be monitored carefully following exercise; carbohydrates may need to be consumed to reverse a fall in blood glucose levels and to prevent hypoglycaemia. There should be an emergency supply of liquid glucose available, and especially in endurance sporting events. If hypoglycaemia does not respond to oral carbohydrates, glucagon can be administered by a doctor, paramedic, parent or person trained in its use. On the other hand, if blood glucose concentrations rise, then extra insulin will be needed.

ARTHRITIS

There are a number of conditions that are classified under the heading of inflammatory joint diseases, of which the most common in children is juvenile rheumatoid arthritis (JRA).

Children with JRA may present with fever, rash, joint pain, liver and spleen enlargement, pleural effusion (fluid in the lungs), pericarditis (fluid around the heart) and may be too ill to exercise, especially in the early part of the disease. Anaemia often accompanies the disease. As these symptoms disappear over time, joint problems become dominant. These may involve multiple joints or only a few, especially the large joints.

The effects of exercise

There are both benefits and risks when exercise is undertaken; a balance must therefore be reached. Cooperation between the physician, the educator, the parent, the child and the sports/exercise personnel is essential.

The benefits of exercise for children with arthritis include:

- improvement and maintenance of joint flexibility;
- maintenance of muscle strength;

- maintenance of bone density;
- cardiopulmonary fitness; and
- improved self-esteem.

Risk factors include:

- worsening of the disease if the exercise is too intense;
- cartilage damage in repetitive weight-bearing exercise;
- ligament and tendon injuries; and
- risk of dislocation in children with cervical spine arthritis.

Recommendations and precautions

Depending on which joints are involved and the extent of their use, some sports may need to be avoided. These include:

- contact sports;
- trampolining (which involves significant spine movement);
- gymnastics, if the child has arthritis in a shoulder or elbow (and given the significant spine movement);
- basketball and volleyball (given the significant use of the wrists and elbows); and
- jogging and high-impact aerobics, if there are problems in the knee, hip and ankle.

Children with inflammatory arthritis frequently have hydrotherapy as a part of their therapy program. Aquatic sports are therefore popular and unlikely to produce any adverse effects.

HAEMOPHILIA

Haemophilia is an inherited deficiency in which there is a reduced ability of the blood to clot; this causes bleeding disorders in males. The condition may be mild, moderate or severe, depending on the deficiency level of the clotting factors.

The effects of exercise

Although haemophilia does not affect energy levels, endurance or cardiopulmonary fitness, haemophiliacs must avoid all sports that increase the risk of serious internal bleeding, especially intracranial (head) bleeding. For example, haemophiliac children should not 'head' the ball in soccer; competitive soccer is therefore not a suitable sport.

Recommendations and precautions

Although all contact sports should be avoided, most other sporting activities are fine. However, some modifications to certain activities may be needed, particularly in regards to the stability of knees and ankles. For example, haemophiliacs should not perform jumping dismounts in gymnastics.

CONCLUSION

Although very little research has been done in the area of exercise and chronic illness, enough information is available for doctors to make reasonable decisions regarding types and levels of activity for the more common diseases. Above all, parents, teachers and coaches must take a positive attitude and consult with the involved health professionals and exercise specialists to determine the abilities, limits, and positive and negative effects of exercise and sport for the individual child. In addition, sports administrators need to provide adequate variation and modification of their sport to allow safe participation for all children. The child should be encouraged to have a positive attitude towards participating in activity; it is the child's desire to participate that will assist in making exercise and sport a positive experience.

SUMMARY

✓ There is a tendency to over-protect children with a chronic disorder and to discourage or prevent sporting involvement. This is generally to the child's long-term disadvantage, both physically and psychologically.

✓ Cooperative consultations between the child, the parent, the physician, the educator, the physical therapist, the sporting adviser/coach and the sports administrator will generally provide a safe but challenging environment in which the child will be able to grow in stature and self-esteem, and develop positive attitudes to life.

✓ If a child's asthma is well managed, he or she can expect the same improvements in fitness as a child who is free from asthma in response to an exercise program.

✓ The low levels of fitness for children with cardiac disorders are largely due to under-activity, not to their actual cardiac condition.

✓ Children with cystic fibrosis can benefit from exercise programs, provided they adhere to their medications, take frequent breaks and replace their fluids frequently during exercise.

✓ Seizure-related injuries are not increased in epileptics if they participate in exercise. Moreover, exercise and sport can significantly enhance an epileptic's self-esteem. Children with epilepsy should therefore be encouraged to exercise.

✓ Children with diabetes must monitor their blood glucose levels carefully before, during and following exercise so as to avoid hypoglycaemia and hyperglycaemia. Carbohydrate intake and insulin will normally be effective in stabilising blood glucose concentrations.

✓ Children with rheumatoid arthritis should avoid activities that put significant stress on the affected joints. It is recognised, however, that carefully designed exercise programs can improve and maintain joint flexibility, and improve muscle strength, bone density and endurance fitness. Water activities are particularly valuable for these children.

✓ Haemophiliacs, like all children, can benefit from well-designed exercise programs and activities. However, contact sports and activities that involve large impact forces should be avoided.

✓ Most children with chronic health disorders are able to be involved in exercise programs and sporting activities. Some activities may need to be avoided or modified, and the child may need to alter his or her expectations, depending on the physical limits imposed by his or her disorder. Nonetheless, given the substantial benefits to be gained from exercise (relative to the smaller risks of injury), children with health problems must be encouraged to participate in a wide variety of sports and activities.

3

Management of common injuries

Dr John McNee

> This chapter looks at the management of injuries that are particularly common among youngsters who participate in regular exercise.

GENERAL PRINCIPLES

All injuries are caused by loading body tissues or a body part with a force greater than the tissue or body part can absorb or withstand. It is easy to understand this if, for example, a leg is hit with a large stick; this causes macrotrauma. The tissues, skin, bone, blood vessels and underlying muscle will all suffer considerable damage. However, it is not so easy to understand how hitting the leg with a small twig can cause major damage. The force is very small. But, if the leg is hit repeatedly 200 000 times, damage will eventually result. This is termed repetitive microtrauma.

So it is with children in sport. A child who falls on an outstretched arm may fracture bones around the wrist, elbow or shoulder (macrotrauma). A child doing a running sport may sustain injury to tissues if the activity is repeated too often, for too long or with too much intensity (repetitive microtrauma). Both internal and external factors contribute, to some degree, to every injury. Figure 9 shows how to identify the causes of an injury and prevent further damage.

Figure 9 Internal and external factors that cause injury

Internal factors	External factors
Body type	Shoes
Fitness levels	Surfaces
Growth status	Environment
Muscle activity	Equipment
	Weather
	Type/velocity of movement

Body type includes body structure, genetic factors and biomechanical function.

Fitness levels with respect to injury are generally related to flexibility of the muscles, ligaments and tendons, and to body strength, cardiovascular fitness and medical conditions.

Growth status refers to the stage of bone and muscle development during growth phases. There may be imbalances between the growth plates (epiphyses), as different tissues and different parts of the body grow at different rates.

Muscle activity relates to whether, for example, a muscle has been conditioned for a particular activity—that is, whether it is trained.

Type of movement refers to such factors as acceleration and deceleration forces, turning movements and the coordination of different muscles.

Velocity of movement is related to forces generated by increasing the speed of motion.

Children's sport should be fun and free of pain. The slogan 'No pain, No gain' should NOT apply to children in sport.

THE IMMATURE SKELETON

Bones grow from special areas called epiphyses, or growth plates. Because these growth plates consist only of cartilage and cells, and lack the minerals (calcium and phosphorus) that give bone strength, they are relatively weaker than the rest of the bone, especially during those times of rapid bone growth (that is, in infancy or during puberty). Epiphyses in the long bones (limbs) are at the ends of the bones, near the joints where the ligaments are attached. If excessive force is applied to the ligaments, tendons, and epiphyses, either as acute macrotrauma or repetitive microtrauma, the area that is most likely to be injured is the weakest area and that is the growth plate. Many fractures therefore occur at these sites.

Fractures to the growth plates are called Salter-Harris fractures and generally need to be treated by a doctor experienced in paediatric fracture care.

There is one other important growth characteristic to be considered in the immature skeleton—the apophyses. An apophysis is a specialised growth plate in a bone where a muscle tendon is attached. These tendons are from the larger muscle groups. Because large muscles are capable of developing large forces or are involved in a very frequent movement, they need to attach to a large surface area of bone. The bone therefore has this specialised area (the apophysis), which, while it is developing, may be subject to considerable stress and, possibly, damage. This occurs especially at the beginning of puberty, when the bones of the limbs are growing rapidly, and at mid-puberty, when the pelvis grows rapidly.

Most injuries to the apophyses are due to repetitive impact, which causes inflammation, or apophysitis. Around the pelvis, where very large and strong muscles attach, the apophysis may be pulled off the main bone, causing an avulsion fracture.

HEALING AND REHABILITATION

All injured or damaged tissue will proceed through the following process of healing:

1 The exudative phase, which is associated with pain and swelling.
2 The macrophagic phase, where repair cells enter the tissue.
3 Neovascularisation, where new blood vessels carrying nutrients develop in the damaged tissue.
4 Remodelling—that is, the laying down of new tissue (collagen) to heal the damaged area.
5 Consolidation, where new tissue assumes the strength and flexibility of the original tissue.

The repair process is likely to be more rapid in younger tissue, but there is no evidence that different types of exercise will speed up or slow down the rate of healing. However, exercise of the tissue, if it is ligament, muscle or tendon, will develop the consolidation phase more completely. Moreover, use of RICE (Rest, Ice, Compression and Elevation) in acute injuries will shorten the exudation phase and will thus help in cell migration and vascularisation. The injured area should be rested. Ice packs (preferably wrapped in a wet cloth to avoid burns to the skin) should be applied for 30–40 minutes and then repeated every two to three hours for 48–72 hours, depending on the severity of the bruising or sprain. A compression bandage will also help to reduce the swelling and bruising, as will elevation if a limb has been injured. Rehabilitation programs should include the following:

- accurate diagnosis;
- detection of the causes of the injury;
- structural repair;
- functional rehabilitation;
- sports-specific rehabilitation; and
- prevention of re-occurrence.

Each of these factors is important in returning the young athlete back to activity.

For the remainder of this chapter, specific injuries will be discussed according to sections of the body.

INJURIES TO THE SPINE

Injuries to the spine may involve the cervical (neck), thoracic (mid-back) or lumbar (lower back) regions and pain may result from acute injury (macrotrauma), repetitive/chronic injury (microtrauma) or from no apparent trauma.

Acute (macrotrauma) injuries

Injuries to the neural cord/cervical spine (neck)
Sports that have a relatively high incidence of injuries to the neck include rugby league and rugby union, Australian

Rules football, diving, gymnastics, boxing, trampolining, horseback riding and downhill skiing.

Injuries to the neck are often accompanied by:

- head injury, including concussion and unconsciousness;
- pain radiating into the arms, hands and fingers; and
- pins and needles, or numb feelings in the arms, hands and fingers.

Spinal cord damage has to be suspected if these symptoms are present.

First-aid must include:

- stabilising the neck (with a collar or sandbags) before moving the child off the field;
- carrying the child carefully in a prone position—preferably on a stretcher;
- rapid assessment by a medical officer or experienced first-aider; and
- careful transport to the hospital or other facility for more detailed investigations (X-rays, scans, etc.).

Injuries to discs

Discs are the compressible cushions between the bones in the spinal cord. Although they are less commonly injured in children than in adults, injuries do occur in the upper and lower back. The sudden onset of pain and stiffness, with increasing pain on coughing, sneezing and bending, and any pain, pins and needles or numbness in the leg, foot or toes, indicates that there is nerve compression in the spinal nerve roots (sciatic symptoms). X-rays and special scans may be necessary to confirm the diagnosis.

Soft tissue injuries

Ligament strain of intervertebral joints and sacro-iliac joints, muscle haematoma (bruising) and muscle sprains are relatively common and may produce immediate pain and lack of proper function. Such injuries heal quickly in children, and the pain is usually not severe or prolonged. RICE and anti-inflammatory treatment is usually all that is needed, and the child is usually able to resume activity within one to three weeks. If pain and dysfunction persist longer than that, then the child should be seen by a doctor or physiotherapist.

Repetitive (microtrauma) injuries

Stress fractures

Repetitive microtrauma injuries of the spine occur most commonly in the lumbar (lower) spine and involve bone damage. The most common part of the vertebra that is damaged by repetitive microtrauma is the arch in the section between the superior and inferior facets. This section is called the *pars interarticularis* (commonly known as the 'pars'). Repetitive arching of the lumbar spine with rotation causes forces of varying magnitude and direction to impinge on that particular section of the arch, which results in bone stress. As in all situations of bone stress, there is a continuing breakdown of the bone until pain develops. The process may continue until full bone fracture occurs. This is called spondylolysis. It may occur on one or both sides of the vertebra and usually involves the two lowest vertebrae (L4 and L5). If the fractures occur on both sides, the heavy vertebral body, which has no support, can slip forward. This is known as spondylolisthesis, or slippage of the spine. If slippage of the body of an affected vertebra does occur, this may lead to future damage of the intervertebral discs and the facet joints, and will cause ongoing pain and disability.

Pars stress fractures develop usually in the early stages of puberty, but may occur in younger children before puberty in sports where intensive repetitive actions occur, such as in gymnastics.

Stress fractures of the spine must be suspected if chronic lower back pain is present. Ligament or muscle strains heal quickly in children (within days or a few weeks), so any pain that remains for weeks or months is not associated with damage to soft tissue (such as muscles, ligaments or tendons); it is more likely to be associated with bone damage.

X-rays will only be useful once a full bone fracture has occurred. If slippage of the spine has occurred, a CT scan may be necessary to assess the degree of slippage.

Management of stress fractures of the spine

- Cease activity for six to eight weeks if there is no bone defect, and for three to six months if a bone defect is present.
- If pain is severe, use a lumbar brace to reduce back extension. In some situations, this may also aid bone healing.
- Follow an exercise program aimed at correcting any specific muscle weaknesses while also strengthening and increasing the flexibility of the lumbar spine, pelvis and hips.
- On return to the activity, change the technique used, if appropriate.

Follow-up: Some athletes will require further X-rays or CT scans to determine the extent of healing.

Generally, athletes with pars stress or fractures are able to resume their sport and reach their previous level of involvement. However, the return to activity may have to be a slow, graduated process and may have to involve changing the technique used, so as to avoid a repetition of the same injury.

Non-traumatic back pain

Scheuermann's disease

This condition involves damage to the growth plates in the bodies of the vertebrae. It is usually accepted that sport does not cause the condition and that it is probably an inherited genetic problem.

Whatever the underlying cause, the condition causes pain, usually in the thoracic spine and sometimes in the lumbar or lumbo-thoracic area. Sport activity does increase the pain in some children but decreases the pain in others.

In its full state, Scheuermann's disease involves abnormality in the growth of adjacent bones of the mid-back spine, causing kyphosis (curvature of the spine) rounded shoulders, and tightness of the thoracic and lumbar muscles, fascia and hamstrings.

Management of Scheuermann's disease

- Simple analgesics such as Aspirin or Paracetamol (Panadol) is usually all that is needed for pain relief.
- Occasionally, stronger medication may be required, such as anti-inflammatories.
- An exercise program may help to reduce pain by providing better postural and structural muscle strength.
- Various thoracic braces have been used in some adolescents when the degree of thoracic kyphosis increases with growth.

The condition will settle as growth ceases, and pain will reduce or disappear. In a small number of children the curvature of the thoracic spine will lead to problems in young adult life, and exercise programs may be necessary. Assistance in this area is provided by physiotherapists.

Infections

Osteomyelitis, discitis and tuberculosis are uncommon conditions of the spine in children and young adolescents but must be considered in cases of acute, severe pain in the spine, especially if the pain is present at rest (such as in bed at night), or if the child is unwell, has a fever, or the pain is excessive and there is little or no obvious trauma involved.

Management of infections

Urgent examination, including X-rays and scans, may be required and hospital treatment is usually necessary.

SUMMARY

✓ Muscle, ligament and joint injuries of the spine in children and young adolescents are short-lived conditions. If pain persists, then another diagnosis is necessary.

✓ Repetitive microtrauma, associated with specific types of activity, is becoming more common as children are subjected to well-meaning but excessive training and competitive loads.

✓ Acute injuries, especially in the cervical spine, may be associated with spinal cord or neural damage.

✓ NEVER ignore back pain in the active or sporting child or young adolescent.

INJURIES TO THE PELVIS AND LOWER LIMBS

INJURIES TO THE PELVIS, HIPS AND FEMUR

Acute (macrotrauma) injuries

Apophyseal fractures

The anatomy of the pelvis is shown in Figure 10. The most commonly injured structures are the apophyses—that is, the growth plates of the bones to which large muscle groups or tendons are attached. The injury that occurs is an avulsion

Figure 10 Common sites of muscle–bone avulsion injuries in young athletes

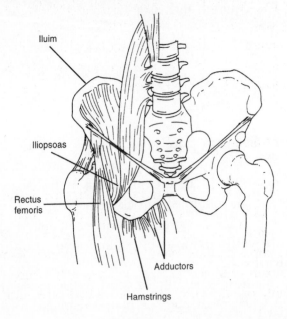

fracture, which means the apophysis is pulled off the main bone by muscle force. These injuries occur as the skeleton is going through its most rapid growth phase—that is, during mid-puberty—as the muscles are rapidly developing strength, and occur in activities involving rapid muscle contractions.

Apophyseal fractures occur with rapid acceleration or deceleration, and result in sudden, severe, sharp pain in the area involved. Movement is limited, because of the pain. X-rays are required to make the diagnosis and to determine the degree of damage.

Management of apophyseal fractures

- If the apophysis is pulled more than 2 centimetres away from the bone, surgery may be required.
- If the fracture is less than 2 centimetres from the bone, the athlete will require six to eight weeks of rest and pain relief to allow healing.
- A rehabilitation program of two to four weeks will be needed to redevelop muscle strength before resuming full activity.

Acute soft-tissue trauma

Hip pointers
Because of the lack of muscle covering the front of the ilium (the hip bone), a fall directly on to that part of the bone can cause injury. This may result in bleeding under the surface bone layer. This injury causes immediate, disabling pain, and an inability to move the hip, or bear any weight, on the affected side. X-rays are required to ensure that there is no fracture.

Management of injuries to hip pointers

- Initial ice treatment plus adequate rest and pain relief.
- Graduated walking activities as the pain level subsides and a return to activity in two to three weeks.
- Adequate padding of the area may be considered during the first two to three weeks of contact sports.

Repetitive (microtrauma) injuries

Stress fractures

Stress fractures of the hip and femur are uncommon in pre-pubertal children but become more common in adolescents as the amount and intensity of training increases. They occur usually only in running athletes, especially cross-country and endurance running (for example, long triathlons). Stress fractures are the result of repetitive loading of the bone from muscle forces, and are more likely to develop where there is some rotational force as well. Therefore, children and adults who have poor bone configuration—for example, those with knock-knees (*genu valgum*), bandy legs (*genu varum*), flat feet (*pes planus*) or pronated ankles—are more susceptible, as are children who have poor flexibility

The pain of these stress fractures initially develops after starting to run, then may develop during the run and remain after. As the condition worsens, pain occurs with any activity, including walking.

Diagnosis of stress fractures is made by a bone scan with X-rays.

Management of stress fractures of the hip and femur

- All running activities must be stopped, and pain relief may be needed for the initial week.
- The bone will heal completely if adequate rest is given (six to 12 weeks).
- Before resuming the previous activity, the alignment must be assessed by a physiotherapist or podiatrist so that abnormalities in running gait can be corrected using exercises or orthotics.
- A gradual return to activity is recommended, so that the loading on the bone is increased gradually. This allows the bone tissue to accommodate and accept the load without further damage.
- Allow sufficient time for the injury to heal before returning to previous activity levels.

Osteitis pubis

Osteitis pubis is an inflammatory process at the pubic joint in the front of the pelvis (the symphysis pubis) caused by excessive stress on the ligamentous joint of the symphysis pubis and the bones of the joint. One common underlying cause is poor flexibility of the hip, pelvic and buttock muscles. Sports where this commonly occurs are soccer, Australian Rules football, activities involving jumps, hockey and endurance running.

Diagnosis generally requires X-rays and bone scans.

Management of *osteitis pubis*

- Reduction of activity.
- Improved flexibility and attention to biomechanics.
- Time.

This condition will sometimes take months to resolve.

Apophysitis

The growth plates of the pelvis and femur are particularly susceptible to repetitive microtrauma. Figure 10 shows the apophyses of the pelvis and femur. Repetitive loading of these growth plates by muscle forces pulling on them causes microtrauma and acute inflammation where the tendon and growth plate meet. This is most likely to occur when the bone is going through a rapid growth phase.

Pain is usually subtle at first, gradually worsening as the activity is continued, and may continue for a short time after the activity stops. There is usually no pain at rest or with walking.

If the pain is bad, an X-ray may be needed to exclude a fracture.

Management of apophysitis

- Usually the athlete will reduce the intensity and frequency of the activity for a period of one to three weeks to allow the inflammation to settle.
- Pain-killers, anti-inflammatories and ice may be necessary.
- Physical therapy includes stretches and a graduated exercise program.

- The activity may resume once the pain has settled.
- There is a risk that once inflammation is present, if the athlete continues the activity at a high level, a fracture may result.

Atraumatic injuries

Perthes disease

This condition involves necrosis (crumbling) of the top of the thigh bone. The cause is thought to be a disruption of the blood supply to the head of the femur, leading to a slow breakdown of the bone. The onset is subtle and not related to sporting activity. However, the first symptoms may occur during running, with pain in the hip or in the knee associated with a limp. It may be thought that a traumatic injury has developed. It usually occurs in children aged four to eight years, but can occur in early adolescence, and is more common in boys than girls. It is interesting to note that problems in the hip will be felt in the knee in young, pre-pubertal children and not felt in the hip.

X-rays will usually show an abnormality of the head of the femur, but occasionally, a bone scan may be necessary if the X-rays do not show any major changes.

Referral to a paediatric orthopaedic unit or surgeon is usually necessary, and a period of restricted activity—and occasionally surgery—will be needed.

Slipped upper femoral epiphysis (SUFE)

This condition is a slippage of the growth plate of the head of the femur and the head is displaced on the femoral neck. It is not caused by activity but, similar to Perthes disease, pain may first be noticed during activity. SUFE is more common in adolescents, and in males than females, and may occur on one or both sides. The underlying cause is not known. The child will usually feel hip or groin pain, but there may be knee pain alone or as well.

X-rays and CT scans are required to make the diagnosis, and surgery is often needed to replace the head, reduce the pain and prevent re-slippage.

An extended period of rest is required, followed by a graduated rehabilitation program.

INJURIES TO THE KNEE

Acute (macrotrauma) injuries

Acute injuries to the knee occur in those sports where there is collision, rapid direction change and high-velocity falls (such as in the football codes, skiing, gymnastics, netball, basketball and volleyball). The anatomy of the knee is shown in Figure 11.

Figure 11   Anterior view of the knee joint (patella removed) showing the anterior cruciate ligament (ACL) and the posterior cruciate ligament (PCL)

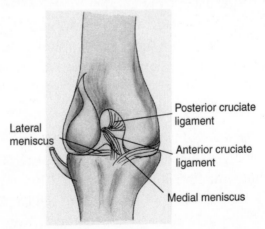

Anterior cruciate ligament

This injury is more common than previously thought. It usually involves a pulling away of the tibial spine, but some injuries will be mid-substance tears, similar to the adult injury.

Frequently, a snapping or tearing sensation is felt at the time of the injury, along with significant pain, and there is usually major swelling within the first one to two hours. The knee is then painful when bearing any weight and feels unstable.

Management of rupture of the anterior cruciate ligament

- Initial rest and ice, possibly crutches to take weight off the knee, and pain-killers.
- Early referral to an orthopaedic surgeon experienced in caring for children with sporting injuries.
- Early operations are now recommended for the majority of children with a rupture of the anterior cruciate ligament. Extensive rehabilitation programs follow to ensure that the child gets back to previous levels of activity.

Posterior cruciate ligament

This is an uncommon injury in children and young adolescents. It usually results from a fall on to the front of the knee or from sudden hyperextension of the knee with force. Pain is the common presenting problem, along with instability, but swelling is not pronounced.

Management of rupture of the posterior cruciate ligament

- Initial rest and ice therapy, and crutches if pain and instability are a problem.
- Physiotherapy referral and exercise program; this injury rarely requires surgery.
- Rehabilitation is usually six to eight weeks.

Collateral ligaments—medial and lateral

Medial (middle) collateral ligament tears are relatively common, while lateral (outside) collateral ligament tears are not. The mechanism of injury is a deformity of the knee: inward bowing in medial, and outward bowing in lateral. These ligaments are frequently torn if an anterior cruciate ligament rupture has occurred, and they may be accompanied by a tear of the meniscus (the cartilage). Pain is usually significant, swelling is not, but the knee feels unstable.

Management of ruptures of collateral ligaments

- Initial rest and ice therapy, and crutches if instability is a concern.
- Early assessment by a sports doctor or physiotherapist should be arranged.
- Surgery is not usually required unless there are other problems.
- A knee brace should be worn for two to four weeks, depending on the extent of the tear.
- Minor tears will heal in three to four weeks,

moderate tears in four to six weeks and severe tears in six to eight weeks.
- Sports-specific rehabilitation is essential before returning to previous level of activity.

Meniscus tears

The menisci (medial and lateral) are cartilaginous plates that sit on the articular surfaces of the tibia and play a crucial role in the function of the knee joint. Injury to the menisci occurs when there has been a rotatory action (twisting) of the knee, such as stepping off, changing direction or landing a jump. Pain is present immediately, especially on bearing any weight, and swelling usually develops slowly over six to 12 hours.

Management of meniscus tears

- Initial rest and ice therapy and no weight-bearing.
- Early assessment of the knee by a sports doctor or physiotherapist.
- Anti-inflammatory treatment and pain relief are important.
- Unless the tear is minimal and heals in two to three weeks, the meniscal tear will require arthroscopy surgery. This will generally require six to eight weeks' recovery and rehabilitation, but will give the best long-term results and decrease the risk of osteoarthritis in adult life.

Note: Fluid on the knee generally means some damage has been caused to the structures within the knee joint and must be properly assessed. Initial treatment should always be RICE (often with crutches to prevent weight-bearing and to relieve the pain).

Knee pains in pre-pubertal children frequently reflect hip problems.

Osteochondritis dissecans

Within each joint in the body, the bone surfaces are covered by a layer of specialised material called cartilage. Damage to this surface is usually associated with pain. If the damage is severe, long-term complications such as degenerative osteoarthritis may result. In children and young adolescents, this articular cartilage in the knees is particularly vulnerable to injury. The damaged area of cartilage may separate or split, and some loose pieces may lie within the joint cavity. This condition is called *Osteochondritis dissecans* (OCD). OCD is accompanied by pain, usually swelling, and often a limp. X-rays with special views may show the loose piece of cartilage or the defect, but often scans are needed.

Management of *Osteochondritis dissecans*

- Diagnosis is essential, so referral to a sports medicine specialist or orthopaedic surgeon is recommended.
- Depending on the extent of damage, the management may be either: rest, with no impact activity for six to 12 weeks; or arthroscopy—surgical removal of loose fragments or screwing the piece back on to the surface. Following surgery, crutches may be needed for six to eight weeks.
- Rehabilitation will depend on the amount of damage, the age of the child and the type of

treatment, but full recovery may take a further six to eight weeks.

Patella dislocations

Dislocation of the patella (kneecap) occurs when the upper leg twists on the fixed lower leg, or when the patella receives a direct blow which pushes it to the outside. There is always tearing of the ligaments that hold the patella in its correct position, especially on the inside of the knee. Often the cartilage at the back of the patella or on the femoral condyle is damaged, as the patella is forced out of the joint (known as an osteochondral fracture). This is potentially serious, as the cartilage is essential for normal function; surgery may be needed to treat the injury.

Management of patella dislocations

- The child, parent or first-aid officer can replace the patella if it does not return to the correct position. However, most will return without assistance.
- Ice, compression, elevation and rest for 48–72 hours.
- Physiotherapy and exercise rehabilitation will be required in all cases, and some will require a patellar knee brace (slip-on guard). This will usually be necessary for six to eight weeks before resuming full activity.

Recurrent patella dislocations

If appropriate and adequate rehabilitation exercises have been undertaken and the patella continues to dislocate, surgery is usually required, such as a lateral release or realignment procedure. These will both require a lengthy rehabilitation period (up to six months).

Repetitive (microtrauma) injuries

Apophysitis (inflammation of bone growth plates)
The two apophyses at the knee which may produce pain are the tibial tuberosity, and the inferior pole of the patella.

Figure 12 shows these apophyses. The tendon involved in both of these is the patellar tendon, the distal component of the extensor muscle mechanism (quadriceps muscles, quadriceps tendon, patella and patellar tendon).

Figure 12 Common sites of tenderness around the knee joint

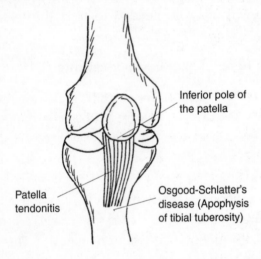

Inferior pole of the patella

Patella tendonitis

Osgood-Schlatter's disease (Apophysis of tibial tuberosity)

The greatest risk of apophyses injury is in the early weeks or months of pubertal development.

Symptoms of this injury are pain on activity (running or jumping, or any sports involving running or jumping), and occasionally a limp because of the pain, and a swelling over the tibial tuberosity apophyses (often referred to as Osgood-Schlatter's disease). This condition is not a disease. It is a common overuse injury, it is benign (that is, there are no long-term complications) and it will recover when the apophysis/bone has completed its growth.

Management of apophysitis of the knee

- Because this condition will resolve itself, the only treatment that is required is for the pain.
- Ice for 20 minutes after the activity.
- Do stretching exercises for the quadriceps muscles and tendons.
- Cease activity if pain is very bad, but generally a reduction in activity is all that is required. The child, and not the parent or coach, should decide what activity is performed.

If pain is on the proximal (upper) end of the tendon at the inferior pole of the patella (Sinding Larsen Johansson syndrome), the management principles are exactly the same.

These conditions are specific to the developing adolescent and are generally minor problems—common, but not serious.

Atraumatic injuries

Patello-femoral disorders

Anterior knee pain is a common complaint among children and young adolescents. This is usually experienced initially as pain in the front or the sides of the kneecap, usually after sporting activities; but it may also occur on walking up or down steps, running on or (worse) down hills, or on sitting for long periods, such as when driving in a car or sitting in a cinema (called 'movie-goer's knees'). The young person finds it hard and painful to squat or bend the knees, and sporting activities such as running distances, jumping and hurdling exacerbate the pain. It may not be painful while doing short-distance running, such as when playing a game of football or netball.

Examination shows no abnormality of the knee joint (that is, the femoral-tibial joint), but there is pain on examination of the patello-femoral joint.

There are a number of types of the condition, but they all relate to the same problem—inflammation of the cartilage covering the back of the patella (retropatellar osteochondritis). The cartilage becomes swollen, then blisters, and proceeds to crack and roughen. The causes are usually due to malalignment syndrome—that is, a variation of the structural alignment from the hip, through the femur, knee and tibia, to the ankle and foot. Such structural variations as femoral anteversion, knock-knees, bow-leggedness, ankle pronation and flat-feet may cause the patella to move (track) in an abnormal path over the femoral groove. The patella may be high (patella alta), or may be tilted laterally. Often the curves on the back of the patella may be shallow, and this may predispose the child to patellar dislocations or subluxations, as well as anterior knee pain.

Management of patello-femoral disorders

- In general, a sports doctor or sports physiotherapist should be consulted to confirm the diagnosis and supervise the management.

- Exercise which involves stretching the quadriceps, hamstring muscles and the ilio-tiboal band (ITB), pelvic control exercises, taping of the patella and, if necessary, orthotics and correct footwear may be advised.

In most children, the above measures will correct the function and movement of the patella. But, of course, the underlying structural variation of bones will remain; this is genetically determined and no treatment can change the shape, only the function. The pain will reduce and then go in most children. However, in some children the pain will not disappear, and a surgical procedure called lateral release may be necessary. This will allow the patella to sit correctly.

In some cases, the pain returns at a later time; as the child grows, the function may change and the pain returns. A further program of exercises and taping, and a change of orthotics, may be required.

INJURIES TO THE LEG AND FOOT

Acute (macrotrauma) injuries

Fracture/dislocation of ankle joint
Because the ankle joint is formed by three bones—the fibula, the tibia and the talus—which are connected by a complex system of ligaments, dislocations of the ankle joint frequently involve fractures of one or more of the bones. If such fractures are found, the bones at the knee also need to be checked, as often proximal fibular fractures may be present.

Management of macrotrauma injuries

These fractures/dislocations are difficult to manage and require attention from an orthopaedic specialist. Very intensive rehabilitation is required for normal function, and a further period of sports-specific rehabilitation before return to sport is considered.

Soft tissue injuries of the ankle

One of the most common acute injuries in sport is the 'sprain' of ligaments in the ankle joint. All sports that involve running or jumping actions are likely to include this injury, but especially if there are rapid rotations as well—for example, netball, soccer, football, squash, tennis and the martial arts. The ligaments provide the static stability of the joint and limit the range of active movement. If that limit of movement is exceeded, the ligaments will be stretched beyond their functional strength and damage will occur. The degree of damage is graded as follows:

Grade I: microtears within the substance of the ligament.
Grade II: macrotears involving a significant proportion of ligament fibres.
Grade III: macrotears involving all or most of the fibres.

All of these injuries are acute, accompanied by pain, swelling and instability (unable to bear weight without 'give'). Children often describe a 'tearing' sensation as they twist the ankle. Inversion injuries (rolling out on the ankle) are the most common. These may be accompanied by damage to the peroneus tendons on the lateral aspect of the joint.

Management of soft tissue injuries of the ankle

- Accurate diagnosis is important.
- Immediate RICE treatment—ICE (ice, compression and elevation) to continue usually for 48 hours. NEVER heat an acutely injured ankle or any other body joint, as this increases bleeding and slows the healing process.
- It is recommended that children be assessed by a sports doctor or physiotherapist, because there is always a risk of injury to the distal epiphysis of the tibia or fibula (Salter-Harris fracture type I).
- Anti-inflammatory management (medication, local gel application, ultrasound and pain relief are important.
- In the first two to three days, crutches may be necessary but the limb should NEVER be immobilised in a cast.
- As the acute inflammation settles, an exercise program should begin. This maintains joint mobility, aids in the healing of the damaged ligaments and helps to prevent a complication called reflex sympathetic dystrophy, which may delay recovery for several months.
- Recovery periods:
  Grade I: two to four weeks.
  Grade II: six to eight weeks.
  Grade III: eight to 12 weeks.

Complications of ankle strain injuries
In some **Grade III injuries**, the ligaments are completely ruptured and healing will not occur or will be incomplete.

This leads to a chronic instability and an ankle that 'goes over' with minimal events and even with no cause—the so-called weak ankle. These ankles may require bracing for sport, and some will need surgical reconstruction of the ligaments.

With **talar dome fractures**, at the time of the injury—when the ankle twists and rolls—the bones of the joint collide and compress. Because the force as the foot lands is directed downwards, the talu is the vulnerable bone and the articular cartilage on its surface (the osteochondral) is damaged and the bone matrix is compressed and fractures. This injury is frequently not seen on X-rays and requires scans to determine its presence and its degree. Some will heal but take several months; the more serious ones will require surgery.

Repetitive (microtrauma) injuries

Because most sports and exercise activities involve running as a part of the activity, stress injuries to the lower limb and foot are the most common chronic repetitive injuries.

Stress fractures occur in the tibia, fibula, navicular, cuneiform bones and metatarsal shafts. The stress fracture is felt as pain after the activity, then as pain during the activity, and then as pain with walking or at rest as the fracture worsens.

Management of stress fractures of the lower limb and foot

- Diagnosis is made by bone scan, and sometimes an X-ray or CT scan may be required to judge the degree of damage or as a follow-up for healing.

- Active rest is required. The child must cease the activity that is producing the injury for a period of time to allow the bone to heal (NOT just to be pain-free). The child can do non-running/jumping/dancing activities such as swimming or cycling.

- Because the underlying problem may be associated with malalignment (that is, a variation from the normal skeletal structure), a biomechanical assessment should be done by a sports doctor, physiotherapist or podiatrist to determine the abnormality and to develop a program to correct the functions and stop the stress problem from redeveloping.

Special considerations in stress fractures

Navicular stress fractures are common in children and adolescents who have *pes cavus* (a high arch) and who do activities involving being on their toes such as sprinters, jumpers and dancers. These navicular stress fractures frequently fracture into or through the bone and will require cast immobilisation for six to 12 weeks on crutches, or surgery. Biomechanical assessment is necessary and most will need orthotics.

Shin splints

Shin splints commonly describe an overuse injury resulting in a painful inflammatory condition along the shaft of the tibia, usually on the medial (inside) border, but occasionally on the anterior (front) border. It is associated with ballistic activities (running and jumping) and is due to muscle forces acting on the bone into which the muscle inserts. The muscles that commonly cause the problem are the soleus in the back of the calf, the *flexor hallucis longus* and *tibialis posterior* in the deep calf compartment. The causes of shin splints are lack of flexibility, malalignment of the bony structures (especially ankle pronation and *pes planus*), excessive activity and inappropriate footwear and running surfaces.

Management of shin splints

- Reduce activity levels.
- Commence flexibility drills and massage.
- Biomechanical function should be assessed and possibly orthotics prescribed.
- Get advice on appropriate footwear.

Soft tissue repetitive injuries

Apophysitis

The two most common apophyses that are affected are the calcaneus apophysis on the posterior aspect of the os calcis or heel bone (the attaching tendon is the Achilles tendon), and the apophysis of the fifth metatarsal on the outside of the middle of the foot (the attaching tendon is the peroneus brevis).

Management of apophysitis of the heel

- These conditions are benign and will recover when the apophysis matures.

- There is generally no reason for the child to cease activities unless the pain is very severe.
- Ice packs used after activities will reduce the pain.
- Stretching exercises may help to reduce the severity of the pain.

SUMMARY

✓ Chronic overuse injuries are common in the legs, ankle and feet in children and young adolescents.

✓ Many are due to poor flexibility and to malalignment of bones.

✓ The best method of treatment is prevention. This can be accomplished by coaches in all sporting activities making warm-up and appropriate stretching mandatory for all children and young athletes.

✓ Biomechanical assessment by sports doctor, physiotherapist or podiatrist is important in the management of all chronic overuse injuries.

INJURIES TO THE UPPER LIMBS

As in lower limb injuries, knowledge of the ages of appearance and closure of epiphyses (growth plates) is important in correct diagnosis of the multiplicity of unique injuries that occur in child and young adolescent athletes. The function of the shoulder (scapula, humerus and the ligaments, tendons and muscles) is complex. The shoulder structure is designed for movement. Stability is provided by the coordinated function of all components, including the muscles that control the scapula as it moves on the posterior ribs.

Acute (macrotrauma) injuries

Bone fractures of the clavicle

Falls directly on to the shoulder or the outstretched arm are the common causes of fractures of the clavicle. Most fractures occur in the mid-shaft, and the fractured bone edges are minimally displaced. Pain over the acromo-clavicular joint is rarely an injury to that joint (as it may be in adults) but generally means a fracture of the distal end of the clavicle.

Management of bone fractures of the clavicle

- X-rays are necessary to diagnose definitively and assess the deformity.
- Administer pain relief and wear the arm in a sling for a few days until the pain has subsided.
- Most clavicle fractures will heal in three to four weeks and do not need other treatments.
- The old treatment of figure-of-eight bandages is not considered to be necessary and may cause more pain.

Bone fractures of the humerus

Fractures at the upper end of the humerus are usually the result of a fall on the outstretched arm, often with external rotation; these are uncommon in children but more common in adolescents. Fractures at the lower end at the elbow (a supracondylar fracture) are far more common in children and are caused by falls on to an outstretched hand or directly on to an elbow.

Immediate pain, swelling and deformity at the elbow is the clinical sign of a supracondylar fracture. The complication that must be checked for is damage to the nerves and blood vessels within the elbow, as this will produce major disruption to the function of the forearm and hand.

Management of bone fractures of the humerus

- X-rays are essential for diagnosis.
- If there is no dislocation of the elbow, the fracture can be treated conservatively in a collar-and-cuff bandage for three to four weeks, followed by an exercise rehabilitation program.
- If there is displacement of the fracture or joint dislocation, then manipulation under anaesthetic or surgical intervention will be required. Referral must be made as soon as possible for orthopaedic management.
- Physiotherapy and rehabilitation will be required in all cases after healing has occurred.

Shoulder dislocations/subluxations

Most dislocations occur to the front of the joint. These are relatively uncommon in children. If they occur, they usually do so in children who have loose ligaments and then there may be only partial dislocation (subluxation). These injuries become more common through puberty, as interacting forces, especially in contact and collision sports, increase due to increasing body mass. Football, hockey, falls in horse riding, and gymnastics are some of the sports in which dislocations can occur.

Dislocations: The ligamentous capsule around the shoulder joint is torn. The rotator cuff tendons over the ligaments may also tear (especially the more anterior tendons—the subscapularis, the supraspinatus and the tendon of the long head of biceps). There may also be bone damage. When the head of the humerus strikes the glenoid fossa (socket), it can injure the glenoid margin or the head of the humerus (called a Hill-Sachs injury). There may be nerve and blood vessel damage, but this is rare.

Management of shoulder dislocations

- Immediate replacement of the dislocation should be done if spontaneous replacement has not occurred.
- X-rays will be needed to determine bone damage.
- A sling should be worn to rest the shoulder, and analgesics and anti-inflammatories should be used.
- Referral to a physiotherapist is usually recommended.
- Children and adolescents under 17 years of age with a full dislocation have a virtual 100 per cent chance of further dislocation, and it is now recommended that surgical repair of the torn ligamentous capsule be performed to get the best possible results.
- Rehabilitation with an exercise program is essential before returning to sport.

Subluxations (partial dislocations): These instances of only partial dislocation are the result of having excessive movement of the ligamentous capsule. This may involve part or all of the capsular ligaments and is usually a congenital abnormality. It produces excessive movement of the head of the humerus in the glenoid fossa and the subluxation may occur with minimal activity. Some children have such a degree of laxity that they can voluntarily sublux the joint. If the laxity is in all directions, it is called multi-directional instability. In some sports such as competitive swimming and throwing sports that require extensive training, the instability can be the result of repetitive microtrauma to the ligaments. This situation causes inflammation of the rotator cuff tendons and abnormal scapular movement resulting in impingement—the so-called swimmer's shoulder. Repeated subluxations with multi-directional instability is difficult to manage.

Management of partial dislocations

- Anti-inflammatories, pain relief, and reduction or cessation of the problematic sporting activity may be required.
- Extensive exercise rehabilitation under the supervision of a sports physiotherapist will be necessary. This will improve the strength of the external muscle groups and help control scapular function.
- Occasionally, surgery will be needed in these young athletes to tighten the lax capsule (called a capsular shift operation). This will still require extensive rehabilitation and is not always successful.

RADIUS AND ULNA FRACTURES

These fractures are relatively common in children and are relatively easily diagnosed. Management with cast immobilisation is standard. Damage to the epiphyseal plates must always be suspected and must be treated, usually by an orthopaedic surgeon or a doctor experienced in paediatric orthopaedics. Long-term growth problems of the bone can result if the injury is not treated correctly.

Repetitive (microtrauma) injuries

Injuries to the shoulder and humerus

Overuse injuries of the shoulder occur in children performing repetitive activities, such as throwing sports, pitching in baseball, and gymnastics. The injury involves the upper humeral epiphysis, and there is widening and separation and sometimes necrosis of the humeral head. It is caused by too much throwing and poor technique at the stage of growth and development.

Management of injuries to the shoulder

- Cease all throwing, pitching and gymnastics until healing occurs—this may take three to six months.
- Shoulder function should be assessed and muscle weakness and imbalance corrected.
- The technique of the activity may need to be corrected.
- On return to the activity, there should be a reduction in intensity, such as limitation of the number of throws or pitches, or a change of routine in gymnastics.

Rotator cuff tendons or 'swimmer's shoulder'

'Swimmer's shoulder' is a common overuse injury in young swimmers. It is due to a relative weakness and imbalance in the rotator cuff tendons and muscles from the scapula (the shoulder blade). These four muscles, with the biceps' long head tendon, stabilise the shoulder joint during movement, aiding the ligaments in preventing dislocation. Especially if there is ligamentous laxity (either congenital or acquired from overuse), these tendons have to provide greater control when acceleration or deceleration forces are applied. The tendons become inflamed (and therefore swollen and painful, especially when doing elevation and overarm activities) and may tear. Muscles of the neck, thoracic spine and scapula are also involved, so the pain can be in the shoulder, arm, neck and thoracic spine.

While this condition is common in overarm swimming events (freestyle and butterfly), they also occur in throwing activities such as javelin, tennis serving and overhead shots, badminton, baseball and softball throwing. As these latter throwing activities also involve acceleration, deceleration and rotation at the elbow joint, they may also present with elbow overuse injuries.

Management of 'swimmer's shoulder'

- Reduction or cessation of the activity producing the overuse.
- Initial analgesics and/or anti-inflammatories.
- Biomechanical functional assessment of scapulo-thoracic movement, gleno-humeral movements, capsular ligament and muscle stability.
- A specific exercise program for the individual,

depending on what weakness and imbalance is found.
- Return to sport only when the weakness/imbalance is corrected and the technique of the activity is corrected. This may take weeks or months.

Injuries to the elbow, forearm and wrist

As discussed earlier, overuse injuries to the elbow occur in children performing throwing activities—for example, pitching in baseball, javelin, and long throws such as in cricket. Children who perform these throwing activities with a sidearm motion are more likely to get the overuse injury. Gymnasts can suffer similar compression and traction injuries to the throwers.

Injuries occur to the ulnar collateral ligament on the inside of the elbow joint, the epiphysis of the medial humeral condyle, the epiphysis of the radial head, and *Osteochondritis dissecans* of the capitellum of the humerus. The other less common injury seen specifically in gymnasts is stress fractures of the distal humerus, due to the repeated hyperextension ('locking out'). These overuse injuries cause pain, joint swelling, soft tissue swelling and a decrease in function.

Management of injuries to the elbow, forearm and wrist

- Investigations need to be done to determine the injury and its severity. X-rays, bone scans, CT scans and ultrasound scans may be required.

- All injuries need cessation of activity.
- Medial humeral condyle avulsion requires surgery with pinning.
- *Osteochondritis dissecans* of the capitellum requires surgery and removal of cartilage pieces.
- All injuries require intensive physiotherapy and extended exercise rehabilitation.
- Modification of technique, and of the intensity and frequency of activity, needs to be addressed when the athlete returns to the sport.

Salter-Harris type I injuries

The most common overuse injury of the wrist occurs in gymnastics and athletes doing weight training, who hyperextend their wrists. The usual cause of pain in pre-pubertal and early pubertal athletes is Salter-Harris type I injury to the distal radial epiphysis. X-rays will show a slight widening of the epiphyseal plate, and a bone scan will show excessive uptake. This is an important diagnosis. If the activity continues and the epiphyseal damage becomes permanent, growth of the distal radius will stop and there will be anatomical and functional abnormality of the wrist.

Management of Salter-Harris type I injuries

- Cease the activity until the epiphysis repairs (six to 12 weeks).
- Reduce the intensity and frequency of the activity for a further three months to avoid recurrence and possible long-term problems.

SUMMARY

✓ Overuse injuries in young athletes in the upper limbs are generally due to inappropriate frequency or intensity of training loads. Strict adherence to correct techniques can reduce the incidence as well.

✓ Modification of activities (such as the number of pitches in baseball, the number of throws in throwing sports, reduction in serving practice in tennis, reduction of numbers of laps in swimmers) will all aid in prevention of these injuries.

✓ Early and correct diagnosis and treatment of upper limb injuries will decrease the risk of long-term complications.

4

Training for speed, endurance and flexibility

David Jenkins and Peter Reaburn

 This chapter looks at ways to develop speed, endurance and flexibility.

SPEED TRAINING

Speed is the ability to move quickly between two places. Depending on the event or activity in which it is used, speed involves reaction time, acceleration, maximum speed and speed endurance. Each of these components of speed can be trained, but first the coach, teacher or parent must decide which components are important. It is most important that the type of speed which needs to be improved is carefully analysed. For example, the drills which can potentially improve the speed of a track sprinter are generally different to those drills which are most effective for improving the speed of games players (for example, footballers, netballers, etc.).

Speed training for youngsters who are yet to reach their teenage years should be restricted to activities such as relays and practice games. Only when a child becomes a teenager will he or she be receptive to more specific techniques for improving speed. For this reason, the following sections on speed will primarily address the procedures capable of improving speed in the pre-adolescent teenager, rather than the child.

The physiology of sprint exercise: Comparing teenagers and adults

There are two important differences between teenagers and adults with respect to sprinting: first, the teenager has less muscle (relative to his or her size); and second, the teenager has a reduced ability to produce energy via anaerobic glycolysis (that is, the 'lactate' system). The smaller muscle mass of the teenager is likely to limit his or her potential to improve power, while the lower anaerobic capacity means that more energy during sprints will have to come from aerobic metabolism and less from anaerobic glycolysis. In practice, this means that endurance training will have greater benefit for pre-adolescents than for adults during sprints. In addition, levels of lactic acid in the muscle and blood will be lower for pre-adolescents following a sprint, which means that they will recover faster than adults.

Designing a speed training program

Before designing a sprint training program for a teenager, his or her speed requirements must first be assessed. For example, tennis players will never reach their maximum speed during competition; instead, reaction time and acceleration will be more important aspects. The following questions should therefore be asked before devising a speed training program.

1 **What type of speed is required?** Estimating the average distance that the teenager sprints during his or her chosen activity will determine which components of speed (such as acceleration, maximal speed, etc.) are most important to include in the training program.

2 **Is maximal speed reached during the activity, and if so, how often?** If we consider a track sprinter, then the answer to the first part of the question will be 'yes'. It may also be true for a hockey player or footballer. It is likely that a hockey player or footballer will be required to repeat a sprint after a very short recovery, whereas the track sprinter, in competition, will fully recover before sprinting again.

3 **If the teenager is not a track sprinter, then what are the movement patterns required in the sprint?** For example, is there a need to sprint in different directions? Tennis players need to sprint backwards and sideways; these types of sprints will require different training drills from those needed for improving the 'straight-ahead' speed of a 100 metres sprinter or long-jumper.

In the case of team players, different playing positions will often have different speed requirements. For example, depending on the field position, the speed demands of an 'openside' flanker in rugby union will differ to those of a wing. Foot and/or body position are likely to change according to playing position. Speed training must therefore take into account special demands on particular athletes and players.

As well as assessing the requirements for an activity or sport, a teenager's strengths and weaknesses need to be analysed. For example, a squash player may be very quick in 'straight-ahead' activities such as a ten-metre sprint, yet he or she may be relatively slow in a shuttle run test, which involves changes in direction. The main point to note is that any training program will only be effective when both the type of speed required and the individual's strengths are carefully evaluated.

Aspects of speed to be trained

As described elsewhere (Dick 1989; Reaburn and Jenkins 1996), there are at least five aspects of speed which can be trained:

- **Reaction time**. Reaction time is particularly important in activities in which there is not enough time or distance to reach maximal speed. Reaction time can be improved with reaction drills (for example, sprinting on a command or a signal).
- **Acceleration**. This is the ability to reach maximal speed in the shortest possible time and can be improved using special drills. The nature of these drills depends on factors such as the intended direction of a sprint, body position, whether the teenager is carrying something (such as a racket), and so on. For example, a goalkeeper in hockey or soccer may practise sprinting from a kneeling position (to simulate the need to get to his or her feet quickly) before moving across the goal mouth to defend the other side of the net. Tennis players may benefit from practising sprints from the front to the rear

of the court (simulating the retrieval of an opponent's lob). Remember that it is important for drills to be specific to common situations, and it always helps if the activity is enjoyable.

One acceleration drill which is enjoyable and teaches both children and teenagers the importance of correct body position and what is known as 'first-step quickness' involves touching several closely positioned cones in succession (see Figure 13). Nine cones are placed approximately two metres apart. The intention is to sprint from the starting line and touch each cone. However, the middle cone has to be touched after each

Figure 13 Sample acceleration drill

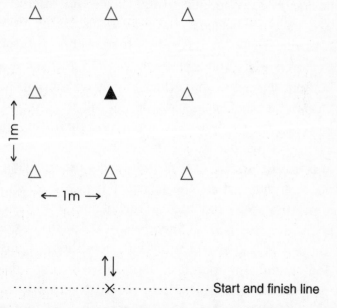

Upon the instruction to 'go', the athlete sprints and touches all the cones. Cones can be touched in any order and only need to be touched once, except for the middle cone, which must be touched once after each of the others. Thus, the athlete must return to touch the middle cone every time he or she touches one of the others.

of the others, so the athlete has to return to the centre before heading off in each new direction. If more than two sets of cones can be positioned alongside each other, two teams can compete against each other.

- **Capacity to readjust balance**. This is the ability to recover or start a sprint from an unbalanced position. For example, it could involve a squash player, having falsely predicted an opponent's shot to the front corner, needing to quickly change direction towards the back of the court. Similarly, a basketball player may benefit from simulating recovery from a minor collision with another player in order to quickly follow a change in play. Balance readjustment can be trained using jumping, balance and stability drills. Shuttle runs, and having to stop sprinting within a certain distance, can also improve balance. Players can also work in pairs, with one trying to push the other over at the start of a short sprint. The skill is to try and recover a good body position and sprint direction as quickly as possible. One particular deceleration drill is called 'stop and go'. Players have to repeatedly sprint, and then stop and go again, on instruction.

- **Maximum speed** can be improved using 'flying' 30-metre sprints, where the teenager begins a sprint from a moving start and tries to maintain good form and speed for 30 metres. 'Innervation drills' (for example, running at 100 per cent all-out pace, then, on instruction, putting in four fast steps) also help to improve maximum speed. Track sprinters (as compared to teenagers who participate in activities that do not allow maximum speed to be reached) are likely to benefit most from these drills.

- **Anaerobic capacity** can be loosely defined as the

ability to maintain a sprint over a relatively long distance (say, 400 metres) or during consecutive sprints, often when the recovery between each sprint is too short for lactic acid to be removed from the muscle. Many team sports are, at least in a physiological sense, simply multiple sprint activities, where time between bouts is too short for the muscle to completely recover. Learning to cope with fatigue is improved through shuttle run activities in which sprints are repeated following a very short recovery.

As stated earlier, boys and girls have lower anaerobic power and greater local muscular endurance than adults. Pre-adolescents therefore recover faster than adults following sprint exercise, which means that when performing multiple sprints, pre-teens require shorter recovery periods than do adults. It is likely, therefore, that children will not show large improvements in response to multiple sprint training

Sports speed

The term 'sports speed' describes the speed required for a particular activity. For example, the type of speed required for tennis differs from that needed for a 200 metres track sprint. The following questions need to be asked before any speed training begins:

- **How important is 'straight' speed?** Clearly this is vital for a track sprinter but not as important for a squash player (who has to move sideways and backwards as well as forwards).
- **Is lateral (sideways) speed and agility needed?** This type of speed is important in basketball, tennis, squash, etc.

- **Is there a need to quickly repeat a sprint?** This is particularly necessary in multiple sprint sports, such as football, hockey, racket sports, etc.

If straight speed, lateral speed and agility are important requirements of an activity or game, attention in training can be directed at improving acceleration, open field running and maximal speed; these are discussed in more detail below.

Most team and individual athletes require good acceleration. However, if we ignore track sprinters for the time being, the great majority of teenagers will only ever sprint over distances less than 30 metres during competition. This means that maximal speed will rarely be reached, and that acceleration plays the most important part in speed and must therefore receive special attention in speed training. Two aspects significantly contribute to acceleration: first-step quickness and correct body position.

First-step quickness is the ability to move in a certain direction as quickly as possible. Often, significant speed improvements over ten metres can be made by eliminating a false step. This is commonly seen when an athlete, wishing to run to his or her right, either rocks back on to his or her left leg, or, even worse, takes a step back with his or her left leg, before then beginning to run to the right. By teaching the athlete to run immediately in the intended direction, with a low, fast first step, time-wasting movements are avoided. As different open field sports require varying start positions, it is essential that most athletes can start sprinting from either foot.

Body position for acceleration is different from the body position necessary for maintaining maximal speed running. While maximal speed running requires a runner to be fairly upright (which allows the legs full range of movement through the hips), the ideal position for accelerating is between 45 and 60 degrees (see Figure 14). If a sprint begins from a standing start (as in, for example, baseball and softball), the angle should approach 45 degrees. However, if the athlete is moving immediately before the sprint (such as running to receive a pass), there is less need for such a low position.

Open field running is where an athlete begins by jogging, but then accelerates rapidly to maximum speed. In football, this sprint may involve a change in direction, physical contact in pushing, being pushed, or breaking a tackle. Factors important in this form of speed are the ability to correctly position the body for acceleration, and the ability to initiate a fast leg turnover. One drill that can train this is called the 'in/out' drill, where an athlete increases speed over, for example, 15 metres, then sprints maximally for a distance of 20 metres. He or she then slows down over a similar distance before re-accelerating and sprinting for a further 20 metres. It is also possible to incorporate changes in direction for improving sideways speed.

Figure 14 The correct and incorrect body positions for accelerating

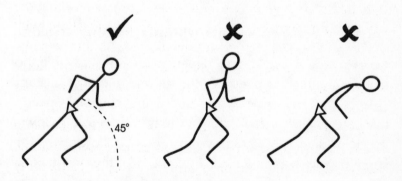

Adults usually reach maximal speed during a sprint at around 40 metres; it can then only be maintained for a limited distance before deceleration sets in. Depending on their age, children are likely to reach maximal speed at between 25 and 40 metres. For most games players, maximal speed will rarely be a determining factor in their performance, and sprint training over distances longer than 40 metres will usually be unnecessary. However, given that some athletes (for example, track sprinters) require speed over 100 and 200 metres, training will need to concentrate on longer distances for some individuals.

Many team players still sprint over distances as long as 60 metres in training and rarely train at shorter distances. This is non-specific when we consider the distances most players are expected to sprint during competition. Of much greater value to many games players would be a run over 80 metres, comprising a 20-metre sprint (acceleration), a 30-metre cruise (open field running), and a 30-metre sprint (re-acceleration). This allows the qualities of acceleration and open field running to be trained to a much higher degree. Game-specific movement patterns and/or directional changes can be used to increase the specificity of the speed drill and ensure a good transfer of speed from training to playing.

Recovery between sprints within a training session

Recovery between sprints depends on how much importance an athlete places on the development of maximal speed. The key issue when improving maximal speed is that the muscles have to be fully recovered following previous activity. We know that even following a brief sprint, it may take at least five minutes for the energy levels in adult muscles to return to normal; bear in mind that, for the same reasons explained above, teenagers will recover faster than adults following a sprint. Remember, however, that if an athlete is forced to repeat a sprint before they have fully recovered, that sprint will be slower—which is not ideal if the focus of a training session is to improve maximal speed.

Occasionally there may be a need to improve anaerobic capacity, or 'lactate tolerance' (particularly when a games player needs to experience fatigue similar to that which occurs in competition). In this type of training, the recovery between sprints is deliberately kept short in order to induce fatigue. It should be made clear, however, that if the child or teenager is involved in several different activities during the week (for school and clubs), then anaerobic capacity will develop quite naturally. Any additional training of this nature may be unnecessary and could easily be counter-productive given the increased risks of overtraining and injury.

Plyometrics for young sprinters

Plyometrics are exercises which develop the explosive capabilities (that is, power) of the muscles; they typically involve a rapid change in direction and high-impact forces. Examples of plyometric activities include bounding and hopping. Clearly, sprinting requires a high degree of power, and many adults who participate in sprint-related sports use plyometric training in their conditioning program.

Although there are some studies which suggest that the benefits of plyometric training are outweighed by the risks of injury, the great number of adults who do perform plyometric training believe that, when used carefully, it can improve power. Nonetheless, specific plyometric training for children is generally not recommended. The main reason is related to the increased risk of injury. As discussed in

Chapter 3, large impact forces can potentially damage growth plates on the bones. This can have disastrous consequences and is a risk not worth taking.

Having said that, some children will perform plyometric exercises as part of their normal training. For example, gymnasts complete plyometric exercises in virtually all their routines, so for this particular group of athletes, specific and separate plyometric conditioning could improve the execution of a range of demanding skills.

One general rule of plyometric training is that the exercises must never be performed while fatigued. Instead, the muscles must be strong and able to cope with the large forces imposed on them.

Strength training for young sprinters

Many athletes require varying degrees of strength for the different demands placed on them in competition. Accordingly, most sprinters undertake some sort of strength training during the year. Correct body position has to be maintained during a sprint, and it is the strength of the abdominal, hip and lower back muscles which are the central elements in adult strength training programs. Strength training for pre-adolescents is discussed in Chapter 5.

CONCLUSION

The type of speed needed in a particular event, sport or game must be carefully assessed before a speed training program is devised. This is critical if the training program is to be both effective and specific. For games players, acceleration is likely to be the most important component of speed; first-step quickness and correct body position are both very important for good acceleration. Recovery between sprints is another consideration when designing a training program. When training to improve maximal speed, a full recovery is necessary between sprints. Alternatively, when training to improve anaerobic capacity, recovery periods between sprints should be kept relatively brief.

ENDURANCE TRAINING

Sports such as swimming, skating, running, triathlon, rowing and most team sports demand some level of endurance. This part of the chapter outlines some of the factors a parent and coach must consider when coaching or parenting a child involved with endurance activities.

Factors determining endurance capacity

Five factors determine a child's ability to be a good endurance athlete. These include genetics, gender, body composition, age, and training.

Genetics
It has been estimated through studies on identical twins that 70–75 per cent of endurance ability is genetic. That is, our parents have given us (or forgotten to give us!) the ability to be an endurance athlete. Our parents have given us a particular body type, a possible 'endurance physiology', a high or low percentage of slow twitch endurance muscle fibres, the ability to recover from or adapt to training stress, and/or the mental constitution for endurance. If we don't have these factors in our favour, we are going to find it difficult to do well in endurance events.

Gender
Post-puberty female endurance athletes generally have a 10 per cent lower aerobic capacity than male endurance

athletes. This is due to the fact that females have smaller hearts which pump less blood and oxygen, a smaller concentration of haemoglobin (the substance in the blood that carries oxygen), and carry greater amounts of body fat than males. While it has been argued that extra fat may lead to better flotation in young female distance swimmers, it is generally agreed that the extra fat found in most females is a hindrance to endurance performance when compared to males.

Body composition

Low levels of body fat are very important to the endurance athlete. No endurance athlete wants to carry extra weight around on a bike, running track, playing field or through the water. However, too much emphasis on this aspect of sports performance in children, particularly young females, may lead to anorexia nervosa or bulimia—both slimming diseases.

Age

Age is a critical factor that influences endurance ability. We have seen in Chapter 1 that endurance (aerobic) capacity is generally stable until puberty in both girls and boys. At puberty, boys tend to increase their aerobic capacity until adulthood, while girls naturally increase body fat levels and appear to decrease their aerobic capacity post-puberty. From adulthood, aerobic capacity declines in non-exercising people at approximately 1 per cent per year, and in masters athletes at 0.5 per cent per year. The main factor explaining this decline is a reduction in maximal heart rate at the rate of approximately one beat per year.

Training

Endurance training improves both the ability of the heart to pump blood to the muscles and the ability of those trained muscles to take up and use the oxygen made available by the heart and blood. Research suggests that training can increase our aerobic capacity by up to 25 per cent.

The trainability of children

Children, like adults, are trainable. In general, they respond and adapt to endurance training in similar ways to that of adults. Children post-puberty, in particular, appear to adapt and respond in similar ways to adults. In contrast, some research suggests that children in the first decade of life may be less responsive to training than adults, even though performance increases.

There are a number of differences between children and adults that need to be addressed. Historically, it was thought that children could not improve their aerobic capacity beyond what occurred with normal growth and development. However, many of these studies were done without following the principles of training, such as overload (making the children work harder over time) or intensity (greater than 70 per cent of maximal heart rate). More recent studies have shown that when children are trained at high enough intensities, they can not only improve endurance performance, but they also show signs of adaptation similar to those found in adults.

A second major difference in adaptation to endurance training is that children appear not to increase their aerobic capacity with training as much as adults do. For example, a 1993 training study on young swimmers showed that, even though the children's aerobic capacity did not improve, their economy improved significantly. That is, for any particular swim speed, they consumed less oxygen. This ultimately means they get faster, despite no increase in the maximum amount of oxygen they can take up.

Objectives of children's training programs

The long-term physical, emotional and social development of children is paramount when developing any training program. Thus, a number of general training objectives are desirable:

- a wide variety of physical development;
- a gradual progression from general development through to specific, specialised training for an event or sport, then, as young adults, to high performance;
- development of the techniques and strategies of the sport or event;
- prevention of injury and the promotion of overall health and well-being; and
- development of the young athlete's training knowledge.

A child's physical development should include training that develops general strength, flexibility, muscle endurance, speed, coordination, and endurance. Once this base level of overall general fitness is developed, the younger athlete can begin to specialise in a sport, or an event or discipline within a sport, at a later age.

Training principles

When undertaking a training program with adults, the effects of training depend on a number of factors. These include:

- **Training intensity**. In general, the harder we train, the fitter we get.
- **Training frequency**. In general, the more often we train, the fitter we get.
- **Training duration**. In general, the longer we train for, the fitter we get.
- **Specificity**. The adaptations to training are specific to the exercise we do.

- **The child's current fitness**. The greater the fitness at the start of the program, the smaller the increase in fitness.
- **Recovery**. If we train too hard, too often and for too long without adequate recovery, we'll get sick or injure ourselves.

Very few studies have been done on children to evaluate the effects of these factors on children undertaking training programs. In fact, few studies have been done on children at all, mainly for ethical reasons. However, the following principles of endurance training can be used when prescribing an endurance exercise program for children.

Safety
Coaches and parents of children actively involved with any form of physical training must ensure safety before, during and after training. These precautions include:

- use of suitable equipment (footwear, padding of goalposts, ovals in good repair, mouthguards, protective equipment such as shin pads or helmets, etc.);
- a suitable playing surface (no holes or exposed sprinkler heads in oval, posts padded or made of cardboard, people and large objects well away from the field, adequate lighting, etc.);
- reduced risk of heat injury (reduced playing time, correct playing attire, drink breaks, lower exercise intensity)—see the discussion on thermoregulation on page 18 for more on this factor as it relates to children;
- qualified supervision and a training philosophy that fits with those of the parents and the child;
- a stipulation that an unwell child should not participate in training;

- an emphasis on skill development and technique, along with fun and social interaction with other children;
- awareness by the coach of the other sports or activities the child is involved in, so that the child's training program can be adjusted to his or her needs; and
- a warm-up consisting of light physical activity and stretching, followed by some event-specific drills and speeds.

Progressive overload

A training program should ensure that the young athlete gradually has to work harder. Gradually overloading the body will cause the body to adapt to that new load. This progressive overload can be achieved by increasing the frequency, duration or intensity of training.

Specificity

Training adaptations are stimulus-specific. That is, if we want to get faster for swimming, we swim fast. Thus, the training program should emphasise the specific requirements of the sport and the particular needs of the young athlete.

Reversibility

Training effects are reversible. If training is not done often enough, hard enough or for long enough, then the gained adaptations or improvements will decline.

Adaptability

Training programs for children should be flexible and take into account the child's other commitments (exams, craft classes, other sports, travel, etc.). Moreover, allowances must be made for recovery from hard training sessions, games and competitions; for illness or injury; and for individual growth patterns. For example, a child going through a growth spurt may lose the ability to coordinate, as nerve development may not be keeping up with bone growth or muscle development.

Periodisation

A good coach will have a training plan that includes hard days, easy days or moderate days in a week; easy, medium or hard weeks; and periods of time (weeks or months) where emphasis might be placed on a particular quality such as aerobic work, speed or technique.

Recovery

This principle of training is often forgotten. We as authors believe so strongly in this principle, that we have devoted a chapter to it in this book. In summary, recovery can be done through light work, correct nutrition emphasising carbohydrates, and adequate rest, including a good night's sleep.

If the above principles of training are adhered to, there is absolutely no research that suggests endurance training is detrimental to the normal child.

Frequency, intensity and duration

These three concepts are crucial to any endurance training program. In general, Table 2 can be used as a guideline for endurance development in endurance sports such as swimming, running, cycling, skating, canoeing, or other sports where rhythmic, large muscle group activities are maintained continuously for a length of time.

Table 2 Guidelines for endurance development in children

Frequency:	3–5 times per week
Intensity:	70–90 per cent of maximum heart rate*
Duration:	20–40 minutes at the above intensity

*In general, maximum heart rate is calculated by subtracting age from 220. However, there are enormous individual variations.

Because there is an interaction between frequency, intensity and duration, there is no exact way to train children correctly for endurance. However, from both a physiological and sociological point of view, three to five training sessions a week is suggested, with younger children at the less frequent end of this continuum.

For endurance development, there is a minimum training intensity below which few adaptations take place. Research from adults and children suggests that 70 per cent of maximal heart rate (estimated by subtracting age from 220) is the minimal stimulus for already physically active children to gain endurance adaptations. However, 60 per cent of maximal heart rate may be enough for the less fit, or for children who have just commenced physical activity after an illness or injury.

Duration of training must take into account not only the child's attention span, but also seek to maintain their interest level throughout the session. A well-balanced endurance program will include a five- to ten-minute warm-up, 20–40 minutes of exercise training, and be followed by a five- to ten-minute cool-down.

Factors influencing training intensity and loads in children

Physical training of children demands that a number of factors apart from the training principles above be considered in the program design. These include:

- The time available to train, given the child's other sporting activities, other interests (craft, music, etc.), and school or work commitments.
- The training age of the young athlete—that is, how long the child has been involved in sport in general and/or the sport or activity in question. In general, the greater

the training age, the more quickly the child will adapt and cope with training.

- Biological age versus chronological age—that is, some children aged ten may be well-developed muscularly and cardiovascularly, whereas another child of the same age may be quite immature in these areas.

Research has identified a number of physiological factors that limit the ability of a child under 13 years of age to undertake high-intensity endurance training. These include:

- a greater demand for oxygen than an adult for any given speed;
- a much lower heart blood-pumping ability (cardiac output); and
- a lower blood oxygen-carrying capacity until the age of 14–15 years, due to a lower red blood cell count.

Taken together, the above factors suggest that excessive high-intensity speed training should be avoided in a child's training program, at least until 14–15 years of age. Also, adult training programs that have high-intensity, high-volume demands should not be used with children.

In contrast, moderate-intensity endurance training has been shown to increase heart size, improve respiratory function, and improve maximal oxygen capacity and performance in children. Thus, an endurance training program for children should include moderate-intensity, rather than high-intensity, endurance training.

Training techniques for successful endurance performance

A common practice of many coaches and athletes is to adopt the prevailing training methods of current world-class athletes in their sports. This approach has not only led to many a good athlete burning out, but also has fostered the belief that *more is better*, with 'big mileage' being seen as the key to successful endurance performance.

In a study on young swimmers, well-respected US sports scientist and masters athlete David Costill halved the volume of training being undertaken by a swim squad and found no change in swim performance compared to a squad who maintained twice the volume. This research strongly argues against the belief that more is better. Indeed, the prevailing training research recommends a combination of both quantity and quality as the keys to endurance performance.

Endurance training intensities

Heart rates are commonly used as a means of determining training intensity in both young and older athletes. The intensities we use are based on endurance athletes knowing their own maximal heart rates for their chosen sport(s). While this can be estimated by subtracting age from 220, a coach of a high-performance child might determine maximal heart rate via a small test. This can be done by warming up well, then doing ten continuous one-minute increases in intensity, starting easy, then gradually building until the last minute is flat out. The test should be done wearing a heart rate monitor and be followed by a 10–15-minute warm-down. It is important to understand that maximal heart rate, even within an individual athlete, is invariably different for swimming, cycling, running, rowing, and so on, due to the different muscle masses being used and the different body positions involved in each sport.

Once maximal heart rate has been determined, Table 3 can be used to establish heart rate training zones.

Table 3 Endurance training intensities based on percentages of maximal heart rate

Zone	Name	Intensity
1	Recovery	<65% max. HR
2	Aerobic	65–75% max. HR
3	Extensive endurance	75–80% max. HR
4	Intensive endurance	80–85% max. HR
5	Anaerobic threshold	85–90% max. HR
6	Maximal aerobic	>90% max. HR

These heart rate zones are scientifically based guidelines, but they are only guidelines. As mentioned above, moderate training intensities are suggested for young, developing athletes. Looking at Table 3, this would suggest levels 2–4 for training and level 1 for recovery.

When using these heart rate zones and a heart rate monitor, it is also important to remember that heart rates will be higher when exercising in hot and/or humid conditions. This is due to the fact that when we train in the heat, we may dehydrate slightly through sweat loss. This lowers the blood volume, which results in the heart having to pump more quickly and harder to get the same amount of blood and oxygen to the working muscles. Second, when training in the heat, blood is diverted to the skin to help offload the heat generated in the muscles. Again, the heart has to work harder to keep the amount of blood pumping to the muscles to give them the oxygen they require to maintain speed.

Bearing these considerations in mind, we will now look at each of these training zones individually.

Level 1 is the recovery zone. The important factor here is that intensity is low and duration short. This type of 'training' is useful after racing, after harder training sessions, when the coach or athlete notices that technique is poor, or when the body is telling the young athlete it is time to go easy.

Level 2 is the minimum intensity required to give an endurance training response. The young beginner endurance athlete might start out at about 65 per cent of maximum heart rate, but as fitness improves or the training years accumulate, the intensity required to gain adaptations will increase. The adaptations that occur with this level of training include:

- increased stroke volume (amount of blood pumped per heartbeat);
- increased oxygen transport in the blood;
- increased blood volume;
- increased ability of the muscles to use oxygen;
- increased capillary (blood vessel) density within the trained muscles; and
- improved mobilisation and use of fat as a fuel.

This type of training, together with level 3 extensive endurance training, forms the basis of endurance training for young endurance athletes and should be performed for a minimum of 30 minutes, depending on the event being trained for. Endurance athletes should aim for a minimum frequency of three training sessions per week, with up to five or six sessions per week for the more competitive and experienced young athlete. Swimming may be an exception to this rule, due to the fact that it is not a muscle 'tear down' sport like running or football. This level of training should be emphasised during the preparation phase of the training year or season and never forgotten during the other phases.

Level 3 training is done at 75–80 per cent of maximal heart rate for long periods (hence, extensive endurance) such as 45–60 minutes. This type of training takes place during the preparation phase of training and produces similar adaptations to those noted above for level 2 training.

Level 4 training is performed at around 80–85 per cent of maximum heart rate and, because intensity is lifted compared to level 3 training, duration is reduced. Examples are 30–45-minute runs, or more intense intervals in the pool. Importantly, the intensity is just below 'hurt but hold' anaerobic threshold intensity and is thus 'strong but comfortable'. The adaptations that occur with this training include:

- elevation of aerobic capacity;
- elevation of anaerobic threshold; and
- improvement in economy or the oxygen cost per unit of speed or work.

Level 5 training should be used sparingly in the young athlete, particularly those new to sport, those with poor technique or those who are not physically mature. However, it is difficult to understand how training at large volumes below planned race pace (levels 2–4) can possibly prepare you for racing (levels 5–6). It is therefore important to undertake some training at anaerobic threshold (level 5). Examples might be 15- to 30-minute efforts or interval training (sets of repetitions) of the same overall duration with relatively short rests between each interval. This type of training aims to expose the body to sustained exercise corresponding to the endurance athlete's highest current steady state pace.

During anaerobic threshold training periods, recovery is critical and base training intensities (levels 1–2) should not be forgotten. Recovery can also be enhanced by eating or drinking carbohydrate-rich foods, since both levels 5 and 6 training mainly use muscle and liver carbohydrate as their energy source and supplies will be depleted after such training. The carbohydrates should have a high glycaemic index (see Chapter 6) and be consumed ideally within the first 30 minutes after training, but especially within the first two hours after training.

Level 6 training should be used minimally with young athletes. However, in non-injury-prone, high-performance athletes over puberty who have correct technique and a high training age, level 6 training may be used sparingly. Maximal aerobic training employs intervals with speeds that are greater than planned race pace but with long recoveries. The overall training volume is reduced, but the intensity is lifted, during this final pre-competition phase, which lasts four to six weeks. Again, recovery (levels 1–2) after these sessions is critical. Levels 2–5 training intensities should not be forgotten during this phase. Adaptations that take place with this type of training include:

- increased tolerance to lactic acid;
- elevated VO_{2max} (i.e., maximal ability to consume oxygen); and
- improved endurance speed.

Table 4 shows the guidelines that have been recommended in terms of the proposed breakdown of training intensities for children aged ten or 16 years.

Table 4 Suggested breakdown (percentage) of training intensities for young children

	10 years of age	16 years of age
Level 1	10	10
Level 2	50	50
Level 3	30	15
Level 4	5	10
Level 5	3	10
Level 6	0	0
Sprint training	2	5

Periodisation of endurance training

The art of training any athlete correctly lies in putting the above training intensities together during a week (microcycle), a three- to four-week block (mesocycle) or a macrocycle of 12–16 weeks to maximise training time and prevent overtraining. Hard, medium and easy days, weeks or three- to four-week blocks are manipulated to stress the young body at times and then to allow it to adapt to that stress.

A microcycle of a week might consist of four training sessions with a few days off, but with two periods of easy and medium days. During the base development or preparation phase where we are getting the 'miles in the legs' or 'kilometres into the arms', the terms 'easy', 'medium' and 'hard' might be distances covered getting longer, or intensity levels 2–4 being manipulated and distances held constant. During the specific preparation or mid-season phase, the same easy, medium, hard schedule might be in place, but hard might be level 5, medium level 3 and easy level 2.

A macrocycle for endurance might be a three- to four-week period where a hard week is followed by an easy week, then a medium week. Again assuming four sessions a week, a hard week mid-season might be 2 x level 2, 1 x level 3, 1 x level 4, with an easy week being 1 x level 4 and 3 x level 2. Remember the objective of each phase, but as a rule of thumb increase volume through the early season phase, then lift the intensity and drop the volume during the mid-season and competition phases.

Tapering or peaking

The art of peaking for competition is a highly individual matter but usually takes place during the last seven to ten days prior to major competition and involves a gradual or

111

dramatic reduction in training volume (kilometres) and frequency. Intensity of training should be maintained. A recent study found that older middle-distance runners significantly improved their performance by sharply reducing their training volume while maintaining or increasing their training intensity seven days before a race. This taper method was superior to both a reduction in training intensity and total rest in the week prior to competition. It is generally accepted that the longer the young athlete has been training, the longer the taper can be. However, if training duration has been short, then a 'drop dead' taper of two to three days where volume is dropped dramatically by 50–75 per cent might be recommended.

CONCLUSION

A correctly planned endurance training program that emphasises a moderate fitness base followed by 'hits' of higher-quality training will allow the young endurance athlete to optimise his or her genetic potential. However, because endurance training involves long and sometimes intense training, the training program needs to be periodised to allow for adequate recovery times both within a week and from week to week.

Importantly with the younger athlete, emphasis needs to be placed on technique development, general overall fitness development and prevention of injury, with moderate training intensities the predominant training intensity.

FLEXIBILITY TRAINING

Very few studies have examined the role of flexibility in sports performance or injury prevention, particularly in children. What we do know is that between the ages of six and ten the range of motion about any joint remains constant and there are no differences in flexibility between boys and girls. However, after age ten and up to 16 years of age, girls appear to possess greater flexibility than boys of the same age. This is due to the onset of menstruation and the effect of female hormones on connective tissue extensibility. Because bone grows much faster than tendons, children become relatively inflexible during the pre-puberty growth spurt, thus making them more susceptible to injuries and coordination problems during this period.

Stretching is important before and after training or competing. Not only does it help to reduce the chance of injuries, but it also assists sports performance by increasing the range of movement about a joint. This is particularly important in sports such as swimming or gymnastics, which require a good range of joint motion to allow correct technique.

Muscles, tendons (joining muscle to bone), ligaments (joining bone to bone) and the joint capsule (the tissue that surrounds a joint and keeps the fluid in that joint) of a young athlete need to be stretched after training or competing. If not, they may gradually tighten and both increase the risk of injury and decrease performance.

Flexibility training guidelines

Stretching exercises should be included in any overall warm-up for sport and involve the joints and muscles used in the sport or activity. However, stretching should, depending on the sport, also be an essential component of training. For example, stretching for increased range of motion is essential for gymnastics, dancing or diving, where joints and muscles are taken to their extremes of range.

Basically, there are two types of stretching exercises that can be used to develop flexibility or enhance sports performance—static stretching and ballistic stretching. **Static stretching** involves slowly stretching a muscle or joint longer than its normal length and holding the stretch for a period of time. This type of stretching has much less chance of tearing the muscle or joint tissues and is the most recommended by sports professionals. The guidelines set out in Table 5 are recommended by sports scientists to enhance the flexibility of a joint.

Table 5 Guidelines for enhancing flexibility

Frequency	3–7 times per week
Intensity	Muscles stretched beyond normal length
Duration	Hold stretch for 6–30 seconds and repeat three times

Ballistic stretching uses momentum to produce the stretch. This momentum is generated by bobbing or jerking movements that produce a sudden and sometimes excessive stretch on the muscles, thus increasing the risk of injury. This is the reason why static stretching is commonly recommended. However, it needs to be stated that the most important principle of training is specificity. That is, you train specifically for the demands of the sport or event. Thus, if a sport such as soccer or softball demands ballistic movements such as high kicks or throwing, then ballistic stretching has a role in training and warm-up. Importantly for safety, such ballistic stretching is only done following static stretching, and the extent of the momentum or jerking is progressively increased during a stretching session under supervision of a trained adult.

Sports Medicine Australia's *Safety Guidelines for Children in Sport* and Recreation recommends the following seven rules when stretching to ensure maximum safety in children:

- Warm-up prior to stretching. (Light jogging will increase the temperature of the joints and muscles, thus enabling them to extend more.)
- Stretch before and after exercise.
- Stretch all muscle groups that will be involved in the activity.
- Stretch gently and slowly.
- Never bounce or stretch rapidly.
- Stretch to the point of tension or discomfort, never pain.
- Do not hold your breath when stretching; breathing should be slow and easy.

SUMMARY

✓ The following aspects need to be considered when developing a training program: training intensity; training duration; training frequency; type of training (i.e, how closely should the activity mimic the sport); the child's current level of fitness and the length of recovery needed between sessions.

✓ Exercise programs for children must take into account the time devoted to other activities (craft, music, etc.), school or work commitments. Above all, exercise training must be safe, fun, promote overall health and wellbeing and include a variety of activities.

✓ Before designing a sprint training program for a teen-ager, his or her speed requirements must be assessed and the following questions should be asked before deciding on the final components of the program:

- What type of speed is required?
- Is maximal speed reached during the activity and, if so, how often?
- What are the movement patterns required in the sprint?

✓ Depending on what is considered important for a particular individual, the following aspects of speed can be trained:

- reaction time;
- acceleration;
- the ability to readjust balance;
- maximum speed; and
- anaerobic capacity.

✓ If an athlete wishes to develop maximal speed, then a full recovery between sprints is needed. If 'lactate tolerance' is to be improved, then the recovery time between sprints should be shortened.

✓ Intensity of endurance training is normally structured around the athlete's maximal heart rate. Certain 'zones' are then chosen depending on the objective of a particular training session or training period (e.g., a recovery session or anaerobic threshold session).

✓ Improved flexibility can reduce the incidence of injury and improve technique; at the very least, athletes should stretch before and after training or competition to improve their flexibility. Ideally though, stretching should be practised almost every day, irrespective of whether the child performs other exercises as well.

5

Training for strength

David Jenkins

> This chapter looks at ways to improve strength
> through resistance training.

Adults have long received sound advice relating to weight
training, as a means of improving performance and reducing
the risks of injury. However, the advice available to children
and pre-adolescents regarding techniques to improve strength
has generally been poor and inconsistent. The current position is that carefully designed resistance training programs
will enhance the strength of children and adolescents beyond
that which is associated with normal growth and development. It is also agreed that the known benefits of resistance
training will outweigh potential problems (such as injury),
provided that certain guidelines are followed. Aside from the
physical benefits, resistance training, as with most other
activities, has the potential to enhance character development
and psychological well-being. Although our understanding is

limited, it is reasonable to propose that resistance training can improve the health of the child and contribute to a continued commitment to exercise beyond adolescence. This chapter provides details on how the young athlete can use resistance training safely.

PRINCIPLES OF RESISTANCE TRAINING

The principles of resistance training are individualisation, warm-up, progressive overload, specificity and choice of exercises, and order of exercises.

Individualisation

The same resistance training program should not generally be given to every member of a group of athletes, such as members of the same football team. This is because differences in ability and size within the group need to be taken into account. Biological age (maturity) will vary considerably within a group of pre-adolescents, even if they are the same age. In turn, maturity will strongly influence the extent to which strength improvements occur as a result of training. It may be that only minor modifications to a general resistance training program are necessary to accommodate differences in maturity among a group of children. For example, everyone may perform the same exercises, but the actual weight or resistance to be lifted or pushed will vary between children. It is likely that due to their genetics, diet or involvement in other activities, different children will increase their strength at different rates in response to very similar training programs. As a child gains maturity, so too will his or her potential for gaining strength and, particularly, muscle size.

Early improvements in strength in response to resistance

training often occur despite no apparent change in muscle size. 'Bulking up', which is also known as hypertrophy, is rare for children who have not reached puberty, and indeed is rare for females even after adolescence. This is due to the relative absence of the male hormone, testosterone. Increases in strength in the absence of changes in muscle size have been attributed to changes to the nervous system and are thought to involve increased motor unit activation and coordination and reduced inhibition.

It is worth noting that scientific investigations have shown that strength increases in children may take longer to occur than in adults. Between ten and 20 weeks of training are needed to elicit improvements in strength for children, whereas as little as six weeks can see improvements with adults. This is probably due to differences in the intensity of training (that is, the loads which adults push are generally higher). Nonetheless, although children will not achieve the same absolute gains in strength as adults, their percentage improvements are likely to be equal to those of adults, if not better, at the end of the longer training period.

Warm-up

As described in Chapter 4, the body temperature should always be raised before training or beginning competition; jogging or some other low-intensity exercise performed for several minutes will normally achieve this. During this warm-up, blood flow to the muscles improves and the muscle temperature increases, which makes it safer for them to be stretched. Stretching should only begin once the body temperature has been raised. This should then be followed by one or two specific warm-up sets on a particular resistance training exercise. In total, it is reasonable to devote around ten minutes to warming up before training or competing.

Warming down following training helps to maintain relatively high blood flow to the muscles and skin, and this helps the body to recover its normal temperature faster. In addition, stretching when the muscles are warm (that is, following exercise) allows them to be more easily lengthened, and this is good for improving flexibility.

It is often said, correctly, that a warm-down will increase the removal of lactic acid from muscle and blood; and that it will therefore reduce muscle soreness in the days following exercise, which is incorrect. Lactic acid is not the cause of the kind of muscle soreness that persists often for several days following unaccustomed exercise. Instead, the soreness is due to microscopic tears in the muscle fibres. So, the warm-down will not significantly reduce the type of muscle soreness that can last for some time after an exercise session.

Progressive overload

For any training to be effective, the body, or particular muscles, need(s) to exercise at a level of intensity or duration higher than those it normally experiences; this is called overload. It is important to realise that it is not necessary to exercise to the point of pain in order to cause overload; rather, the idea is to gradually increase the difficulty. In resistance training, this means that as muscles become stronger, the resistance (or weight) should be increased by not more than 5–10 per cent.

When the same exercises are repeated in succession, they are termed repetitions or 'reps'. For example, if a person performs ten press-ups in succession, he or she completes ten reps. If these press-ups are performed without a rest, they are called a set. After a short rest, it is often possible (and desirable) to perform another set of the same exercises. The workload for that particular muscle group can then be calculated as:

Number of sets x Number of reps in each set x
The weight or resistance (load)

When young athletes exercise using their upper body (the chest, shoulders, arms, etc.), they should perform between eight and 12 reps to the point of fatigue in each set. For the lower body (legs), the number of reps within each set should average between 15 and 20. It is also recommended that when a particular exercise is being learned, there need only be one set completed for that exercise. Overload should not be the priority during the learning phase of a new skill. In addition, single sets will reduce the extent of muscle soreness, which is particularly common at the start of any training program.

How can you estimate the load that will cause fatigue at between eight and 12 reps for the upper body and between 15 and 20 reps for the lower body? The answer is trial and error, and you should expect to take one or two sessions to gauge the appropriate load or resistance for each exercise. If and when upper and lower body exercises can be performed 12 and 20 times respectively, then it is time to increase the resistance (that is, the weight or load) by between 5 and 10 per cent. That will bring down the reps into the desirable range. For adults, there is much to be said for varying the number of reps, as variation tends to increase adaptation. However, children and pre-adolescents should maintain reps in the 8–12 and 15–20 range; maximal or near-maximal lifts should always be avoided, due to the increased risk of injury.

Overload can be imposed by increasing the resistance (as just described) and/or increasing the number of sets performed in a training session. If you increase the resistance, you raise the *intensity*; by increasing the number of sets, you raise the *volume*. Either way, overload is increased.

Table 6 Details and examples of basic and intermediate/advanced resistance training programs

Example basic program

Duration: 2–6 weeks

Sets: 3

Reps: 8–12 (upper body), 15–20 (lower body)

Recovery between sets: 3–5 minutes

Exercises:

Leg press

Bench press

Leg curls

Arm curls

Military (shoulder) press

Upright rowing

Sit-ups

Example intermediate/advanced program

Duration: 8–24 weeks

Sets: 3

Reps: 8–12 (upper body), 15–20 (lower body)

Recovery between sets: 3–5 minutes

Exercises:

Leg press

Leg squat

Bench press

Single arm extension

Single arm curls

Single leg curls

Military (shoulder) press

Upright rowing

Calf raises

Sit-ups

Each training session should include one exercise for each major muscle group. For example, bench press for the chest and shoulders would not be accompanied by inclined flies in the same training session (as both exercises involve similar muscles). It is also recommended that in each training session, there should be between six and ten different exercises (see Table 6). For each exercise, there should be between one and three sets. And there should not be more than three resistance training sessions a week. This is because, for children at least, training should be balanced across a wide range of activities. Any more than three resistance training sessions a week will inevitably reduce the time available for other equally important activities, such as running, skill development, team practice, etc. It is important to avoid the situation where children are forced to invest a disproportionate period of time in a given activity from which there is relatively little improvement.

Specificity and choice of exercises

Choice of resistance exercises will depend upon suitability of equipment, complexity of the techniques to be used and the muscle groups to be exercised. Rather than concentrating on one particular body part or muscle group, resistance training for pre-adolescents should be balanced and involve all the major muscle groups. Carefully constructed training programs prescribed by qualified instructors will avoid imbalances and/or tightness around the joints. Above all, activities should be enjoyable and safe.

The most common types of resistance training equipment are 'machines', which typically have wire attached to metal plates, and 'free weights'—bars and disks which can be assembled and dismantled before and after a series of exercises. Some gyms also provide hydraulic and 'quasi-isokinetic' devices.

It is possible to debate the advantages and disadvantages of different resistance training equipment almost indefinitely. Above all, selection of exercises must be decided by the effectiveness, safety and convenience of the equipment.

Order of exercises

A resistance training session can be completed in at least two ways. First, it may be possible to perform the exercises in a circuit. For example, after completing one set (of reps) on the same exercise, a different exercise is performed, then a another different one, and so on. After completing single sets with the whole selection of exercises, you return to the first and go through the lot again—in a circuit. A benefit of circuit training is that it tends to improve endurance fitness as well as strength. However, if a circuit is not possible, it will be necessary to do a number of consecutive sets of, for example, the bench press before moving on to complete three sets of different exercise. Whether or not a circuit is chosen will largely depend on the availability of equipment and the number of people training at the same time. Either way, exercises need to be arranged so that muscle groups can recover between sets; a five-minute rest may be needed between sets for adequate recovery to occur. In terms of when to do each exercise, the same muscle group should not be used in consecutive exercises. For example, if it is decided that the military (or shoulder) press and bench press need to be completed in the same training session, then some other exercise should be performed in between them, such as the leg press. The chest and shoulders can then recover while the legs are being exercised.

RISKS FROM RESISTANCE TRAINING

The most serious injury that a child could receive from resistance training is damage to a growth plate (or epiphysis) which is located at the end of bones. This could impair growth of the bone in subsequent years. Additional injuries can potentially occur to the joint surface and to the point of tendon insertion. However, the current view of the scientific community is that, provided maximal and near-maximal lifts, and overhead and explosive lifts (such as the snatch, and clean and jerk), are not performed by pre-adolescents, and that excessive overload is avoided, resistance training does not present any greater risk to children than it does to adults.

Given that resistance training will contribute to the chronic stress of the musculoskeletal system, consideration must be given to both the relative level of maturity of a child and to his or her involvement in other activities. The coach, teacher and/or parent must be mindful of signs of stress (including overtraining and increased susceptibility to injury); modification to the frequency, volume, intensity and progression of a training schedule may be necessary. Self-improvement should be promoted, rather than competition with other children. Similarly, children must never compete with or train at the same intensity as adults. It is worth re-emphasising that any resistance exercise for children in the six- to ten-year age range should focus on skill development which will promote the learning of movement patterns against very little resistance. Resistance training for children in this age range should comprise only a small component of their weekly range of activities.

Precautions

Everyone, including children, should have a medical examination before beginning any training program. Equipment must be regularly maintained, and the training environment must be safe. Once the child is cleared for exercise, correct technique and thorough instruction must be taught for all exercises. Moreover, instruction must be presented in a way that children will understand. A qualified strength and conditioning coach should oversee the program, and realistic goals, outcomes and individual needs of individual children must be carefully addressed.

Some safety and technical aspects in addition to those discussed above include:

- A joint should be moved through the complete range of motion during a given exercise.
- Exercises should be performed in a slow, controlled manner.
- Breathing should be regular during exercise.
- An adult should always be in attendance during training; the sessions should be supervised.
- When using free weights, there should always be at least one 'spotter'. The spotter assists in lifting the weight should the person performing the exercise be unable to complete a set. The spotter plays a crucial role in making the exercises safe.
- Before using machine weights, check for frayed cables and belts, worn pulleys and chains, loose padding and rough movement of the levers. The equipment should not be used if these problems exist.
- When using machine weights, do not allow stacks of weights to bounce or crash down. If this happens, the resistance is too high.

- When using machine weights, keep hands away from all moving parts, including (and especially) the stacks of weights. Do not try to dislodge a pin that may be stuck when the weights are suspended.
- When using free weights, ensure that the bars are evenly loaded and that collars are used.
- Avoid backing into others.
- Be aware that the bars are often longer than you think; be careful not to collide with them, especially those kept at head height.
- Put the equipment back in the appropriate place following the training session.

Table 7 summarises the guidelines for safe resistance training.

Table 7 Guidelines for safe resistance training

- Gain medical clearance.
- Receive qualified instruction.
- Warm-up before training.
- Use individualised training programs.
- Train with a partner and under adult supervision.
- Check the equipment before using it.
- Train all major muscle groups.
- Exercise the muscles through their full range of motion.
- Undertake resistance training on alternate days.
- Limit the number of resistance training sessions to three times a week.
- Complete between eight and 12 reps (upper body) and 15–20 reps (lower body) in each set.
- Warm-down following training.

SUMMARY

✓ Provided certain guidelines are followed, the benefits of resistance training for children outweigh the potential problems (for example, an over-emphasis on resistance work relative to other activities, the risks of injury, etc.).

✓ Programs need to be tailored to the individual. Blanket programs that fail to take into account differences in maturity, starting levels, genetic predisposition and concurrent activities will fail to elicit improvements in strength and may increase the risk of injury.

✓ Children will increase their strength, but not their muscle size, following a resistance training program. The reason is that they have a relative absence of testosterone.

✓ Children will not gain the same absolute improvements in strength as adults. However, the same percentage improvements are likely. It seems, however, that the duration of the training program has to be considerably longer for children to gain the same percentage strength increases as adults.

✓ Children should be medically cleared before beginning any training program. In addition, all training sessions should begin with a ten-minute warm-up and end with a warm-down.

✓ Upper-body exercises should involve between eight and 12 reps to fatigue, while lower body exercises should involve between 15 and 20 reps.

✓ Each training session should involve between six and ten different exercises. These should be arranged so that exercises involving similar muscle groups are not performed consecutively.

✓ Pre-adolescents should avoid maximal or near-maximal lifts, as well as overhead and explosive lifts. The risk of injuries to the growth plates, joint surfaces and points of tendon insertion on bones will then be minimised.

✓ A qualified strength and conditioning coach should provide effective instruction and supervise all training sessions. The goals of the program must be achievable, and training must be enjoyable. The temptation to compete with others (including adults) during training must be discouraged.

✓ Resistance training must be balanced, in the sense that all the major muscle groups should be trained. In addition, resistance training should not dominate a child's activity program. Skill development and other components of fitness are equally important.

6

Enhancing recovery

Peter Reaburn

 This chapter looks at techniques for enhancing recovery from training and competition.

Parents of sporting children know that the petrol and food budgets are always high. Children who are into sport generally play or train from three up to ten times a week. The same children have school, homework, a home life and a social life to keep them busy as well. All this physical and emotional energy can also make youngsters tired, particularly if they train hard and often. There are a number of strategies that an astute parent or coach can implement to ensure their young athlete maintains their energy levels for work or play and maintains their enjoyment in the sport.

Training sessions in children's sport are designed to bring about improvements in endurance, speed or technique by progressively overloading the young body by stressing the capacity we want to develop. This extra stress often leads to a degree of physical or psychological fatigue. Young bodies adapt to training more quickly when fatigued systems are restored to normal levels as quickly as possible after training.

The process of adapting to training is sometimes called overcompensation. If there is sufficient recovery before the next training session, the body will improve its capacity to cope with that session. The coach or parent who plans recovery strategies for their young athletes not only accelerates the natural adaptations to training by reducing the time it takes for their athlete to reach the overcompensated state referred to in Figure 15, but will also have a happier and more energetic child who is capable of meeting the other demands in their life, such as homework and home commitments.

The purpose of this chapter is to present some realistic recovery strategies that may help your children or athletes recharge their batteries between training sessions.

Figure 15 Fa.̄ er adaptation through faster recovery

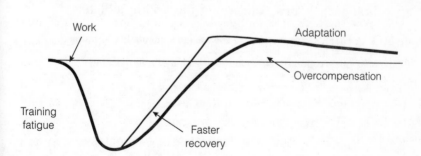

Source: Adapted from Calder (1996).

RECOVERY STRATEGIES

Monitoring overreaching or burnout

If positive adaptation to training leads to improved performances, then negative adaptations can also occur. Overtraining or overreaching by training too hard, too often, or for too long without adequate recovery can not only negatively affect a young athlete's immune system and cause sickness, but can also lead to overuse injuries or psychological burnout when the child may lose motivation or even lose all interest in sport.

The onset of these conditions is diverse and varied. No two children will respond to training in the same way. Adaptation rates also vary from one athlete to another, so it is not always appropriate to prescribe the same workloads for all athletes. It is essential to monitor their responses to training so that workloads can be varied accordingly. Table 8 lists some easily monitored factors that a parent or coach can use to determine whether their child is reaching a stage of overreaching. If this occurs, it is time to meet with the coach and/or others to discuss strategies for enhancing the child's recovery, modifying the training or addressing the psychological issues concerning the young athlete.

Table 8 A coach's observations of the athlete's adaptation to training

Coaching observations	Signs and symptoms of overreaching
Direct communication	Athletes tell me that: • they have heavy legs • they don't feel good • their legs are sore • they are constantly tired
Body language	Facial expression and colour The look in their eyes

Coaching observations	Signs and symptoms of overreaching
	Bending over to recover after an effort
	Bad technique compared to normal
Physiological	Increase in resting heart rate by more than 6bpm above normal
	Loss of body weight (more than 3 per cent)
	Loss of appetite
Psychological	Low motivation
	Low concentration
	Aggressiveness
	No self-confidence
Other	Poor eating habits
	Disturbed sleep patterns (plus or minus 2 hours for more than 2 days)

Source: Guy Thibault (1993), Canadian speed skating coach. Adapted from Calder (1996).

Warm-down

Following hard training or competing, there are by-products of energy breakdown and muscle contraction that need to be cleared from the muscles to enhance recovery. Moreover, the muscles that have been used during exercise will stay in a slightly contracted state after hard exercise and may cause muscle soreness. Thus, a warm-down that includes low-intensity exercise keeps the blood flowing to the worked muscles and flushes them of the by-products, while stretching gets the muscles back to their normal length more quickly.

The best way to keep blood flowing to the worked muscles is with light activity that was the same as the exercise. That is, swimmers should swim for three minutes or more, runners should jog, and football players should jog or walk. Stretching is also essential and should specifically stretch the joints and muscles used in the sport (see Chapter 4).

Sleep

Sleep is a most important form of recovery. A good night's sleep of seven to nine hours provides invaluable adaptation time for young athletes to adjust to the physical and emotional stress they experience during their normal day. Table 9 offers some strategies that may prove useful in encouraging your child to adopt good sleeping habits.

Table 9 Strategies for developing good sleeping habits in young athletes

Things to do:

- Use relaxation techniques before going to bed (listening to relaxing music, reading).
- Go to sleep only when you are sleepy.
- Go to bed at the same time each night.
- Get up at the same time each day.

Things to avoid (evening):

- Caffeine (e.g. coffee, tea, coke, chocolate)
- Nicotine
- High-protein meals (meat)

Source: Adapted from Calder (1996).

Cross-training

Cross-training means doing some other activity apart from just the same sport all the time. Cross-training can often be used as a form of active recovery as long as the intensity is light and the duration short. Pool work, either walking or swimming, particularly backstroke and sidestroke, are excellent modes of active recovery after a game or race and are now frequently used by many elite football teams and athletes.

Rest days

Rest days are essential for all athletes, young and old. At least one day per week should be a non-training day. This allows young athletes time for physical recovery, as well as time to develop interests outside sport so that they can have a balanced lifestyle. It also helps to prevent staleness and boredom. A child with one or two interests beside their chosen sport can provide for this stimulation more readily than the athlete who focuses on sport to the exclusion of everything else. Rest days enable young athletes to maintain a healthy balance in their lives.

Carbohydrate intake

Replacing fluid and carbohydrate stores after training is important for most sports. Carbohydrate loading before an event or training is designed to maximise the storage of glycogen and minimise the onset of fatigue. The right types of food to eat one to two hours before training are those with a low glycaemic index (GI). That is, they are slowly absorbed into the bloodstream of the athlete and can keep their energy levels up while training. After training or racing, the best time for replenishing the used carbohydrate stores is within the first hour following exercise.

It is especially important to eat the right type of carbohydrates following hard training sessions or races/ games, particularly following heavy contact and bruising, such as in football. Muscle damage delays muscle carbohydrate rebuilding, particularly after the first 48 hours. Therefore, it is important to maximise the time when there is an increase in carbohydrate building by providing a high post-exercise carbohydrate intake during the 24 hours after training or playing. The right type of carbohydrate to have after training or competing is one that has a high GI.

The GI measures the extent to which blood glucose is elevated above resting levels for a period of time after eating a food containing 50 grams of carbohydrate. The increase in blood glucose is expressed as a percentage relative to the increase observed after eating a standard type of carbohydrate such as bread or simple glucose, which rate 100. Foods can be classified as having a high (greater than 85), moderate (60–85) or low (lower than 60) GI (see Table 10).

Table 10 Carbohydrates that have a high, moderate or low glycaemic index (GI)

High GI (greater than 85)	Moderate GI (60–85)	Low GI (lower than 60)
Glucose (4.2 tbsp)	Rice (1 cup)	Apples (2.4)
Sugar (4.2 tbsp)	Oatmeal (2.1 cups)	Dates (8)
Bread (3.5 slices)	Pasta (1.5 cups)	Figs (5)
Potatoes (1)	Grapes (3.1 cups)	Peaches (5)
Sweet corn (1.2 cups)	Oranges (3)	Pears (2)
Honey (2.8 tbsp)	Sweet potato (1.3 cups)	Plums (5.6)
Bagels (1.6)	Baked beans (0.9 cup)	Beans (1.5 cups)
Raisins (0.4 cup)		Lentils (1.2 cups)
Watermelon		Yoghurt (2.8 cups)
Lucozade		Milk (4.3 cups)
Lollies		
Weetbix		
Cornflakes (2 cups)		

Note: The figures in brackets are the amount required to yield 50 grams of carbohydrate.

Carbohydrates eaten during recovery should be rapidly absorbed. That is, they should have a high GI. They should also be combined with fluid intake, since it takes about 3 grams of water to store 1 gram of carbohydrate in a muscle. In contrast, usual meals of young athletes should contain slowly digestible sources of carbohydrates and thus have a low GI (for example, cereals, beans and fruit).

Fluids

Monitoring fluid loss during or after training or playing or racing minimises the risks of dehydration and, thus, fatigue. A bodyweight loss of 2 per cent or more during exercise results in a reduction in performance. Educating young athletes to drink in order to keep pace with sweat rates is important, and this can be monitored through urine checks (clear urine is ideal) and pre- and post-training weighing (1 kilogram lost = 1 litre of fluid). For an event lasting less than 60 minutes, water should suffice; but for longer events, isotonic sports drinks (Gatorade™, Powerade™, Sports Plus™, Exceed™, etc.), which help to stimulate the desire to drink, restore electrolyte balances and provide carbohydrate are recommended.

Importantly, young athletes have a reduced thirst mechanism. They are therefore more prone to dehydration than adults. Furthermore, they have been shown to be more likely to drink flavoured drinks during and after exercise, rather than water. This suggests the use of drinks flavoured with cordial, sports drinks or non-caffeine soft drinks for recovery after exercise, and sports drinks during exercise, particularly in hot or humid conditions.

Hot and cold water therapies

Water therapies have always been seen as Eastern European and have been under-used and under-valued in Australian sport. Contrasting hot and cold showers, or using a hot shower with a cold bath, increases the blood flow in the muscles and skin and stimulates the nervous system. Pressure from jets in spas and shower nozzles enhances muscle relaxation by stimulating light contractions in the muscles.

Young athletes need to be reminded to drink before, during and after water recoveries, as sweating tends to go unnoticed in water. Importantly, the times suggested in Table 11 need to be monitored in order to prevent dehydration and nervous system fatigue. Young athletes should feel relaxed yet stimulated afterwards, not sleepy and tired.

Table 11 Guidelines for hot and cold water therapies

How to use:

- Rehydrate before, during and after session.
- Massage skin with soap during the session.
- Alternate:

	Hot (35–38°C)	Cold (10–16°C)
Shower	1–2 minutes	(10–30 seconds) repeat x 3
OR		
Spa/bath	3–4 minutes	(30–60 seconds) repeat x 3

- Shower and rehydrate to finish.

When to use:

- Showers can be used anytime—before, during or after a session.
- Spas and baths are best left until the end of the day.

Source: Adapted from Calder (1996).

Note: Do not use a spa if the athlete has a virus or cold or recent soft tissue injury.

SUMMARY

✓ Recovery is just as important a component as training for the young, active athlete. Warming down with light activity, stretching, high glycaemic index foods, fluid replacement, hot and cold showers, and restful sleep are ideal strategies for young athletes to be encouraged to use, not only to maximise their enjoyment and potential, but to minimise fatigue and possible overreaching.

7

Nutrition and exercise

David Jenkins

 This chapter looks at nutrition for the young athlete.

Health professionals now accept that adult health is strongly influenced by dietary habits developed in childhood and adolescence. A good example is the relationship between osteoporosis later in life and calcium intake coupled with activity before and during puberty. The onset and severity of osteoporosis are closely related to the extent to which bone is laid down during the growing years. In other words, adults can gain a degree of protection from osteoporosis if bone density through diet and exercise is maximised in their youth. Aside from the long-term health implications, nutrient intake during childhood and adolescence must meet not only the demands of rapid growth and development, but also those of any activities in which a child or teenager is involved.

To complicate matters, many youngsters are more concerned with body image and independence than with health and optimal performance. Indeed, Grundy (1994) describes children and adolescents as the most nutritionally neglected group participating in modern sport. This chapter will attempt to address this problem by providing advice on how to meet the nutritional demands of active youngsters. We will review nutritional practices which optimise performance in training and competition and also address weight control and eating disorders.

MONITORING ENERGY INTAKE

Children who fail to meet their energy requirements are quite likely to suffer from fatigue, irritability and poor concentration. It is important to remember that energy intake (that is, calories—or, more correctly, kilojoules) must be sufficiently high to meet both growth *and* exercise demands, and to provide a balanced intake of nutrients. This is easier said than done for active, growing youngsters. As is the case for extremely active adults, the difficulty lies in consuming high quantities of food at regular intervals throughout the day. Three main meals a day may simply not provide sufficient energy. Therefore, snacks (for example, high-carbohydrate fluids, supplements, diluted cordials and fruit juices, etc.) may be necessary to meet a potential energy shortfall. This is particularly important for young athletes who practise or train for relatively long periods of time (such as swimmers, gymnasts, etc.).

Children who have too little energy will fail to recover between training sessions and have difficulty in maintaining or increasing their body weight. Coaches, teachers and parents should watch for such signs and recommend an increase in energy intake (and/or frequency of eating) if they appear. Remember, also, that if energy intake is lower than it should be, there is a good chance that vitamin, mineral and protein requirements may not be met.

Active children should aim to consume between 55 and 60 per cent of their energy intake in the form of carbohydrates, less than 30 per cent in the form of fats, and between 12 and 15 per cent in the form of proteins.

Carbohydrates

When carbohydrate is eaten, the body breaks it down and makes it available to the cells as glucose. Muscle and liver cells take up this glucose from the blood and store it as glycogen, which is the most valuable fuel source used by muscles during most types of exercise. Thus, adequate dietary carbohydrate intake is necessary to maintain levels of muscle and liver glycogen and to perform well. In addition, carbohydrate plays an essential role in providing energy for growth and repair. Inadequate carbohydrate intake can lead to low glycogen (stored fuel) levels in the muscles and liver and potentially reduce the availability of energy for growth. Moreover, low carbohydrate intake before and during exercise leads to early fatigue, poor concentration and a slow recovery following exercise. Pre-adolescents need to eat 7–8 grams of carbohydrate for every kilogram of their body weight each day. (Foods that provide 50 grams of carbohydrate are shown in Table 12.)

Table 12 50 gram serves of carbohydrate

Food	Quantity
Bread and cereals	
Bread	4 slices
Pocket bread	2 average
Cooked rice	1.5 cups
Weet-bix™/Vitabrits™	4 biscuits

Food	Quantity
All Bran™	1 cup
Flakes with fruit	1.5 cups
Sustain™	1 cup
Oats (raw)	0.75 cup
Oats (cooked)	2.25 cups
Fruit muffin	1.5 average
Breakfast bar	2 bars
Crispbread	8 large
Pikelets	4 average
Muesli bar	2.5 bars
Untoasted muesli	1 cup
Crumpet	2 average
Scone	2–3 average
Pancake	2 large
Pasta (cooked)	1.5 cups
Dairy products	
Yoghurt (fruit)	2 tubs
Yoghurt (plain)	3 tubs (600 g)
Milk (all types)	1 litre
Skim milk powder	5 tbsp
Starchy vegetables	
Corn	2 cups
Potato (cooked)	2 large
Lentils/kidney beans	1.5 cups
Baked beans	1.5 cups
Fruit	
Banana	2 large
Apricots	10 medium
Apple/orange/pear	3 average
Grapes	2 medium bunches
Peach	6 medium
Strawberries	3.5 cups
Melon	3.5 cups
Mango	1 large
Dates	9
Apricots	10 whole or 20 halves

Food	Quantity
Sultanas	6 tbsp
Fruit salad	2 cups
Tinned fruit	2 cups
Fruit snack pack	3
Miscellaneous products	
Honey/golden syrup/jam	2 tbsp
Fruit Roll-up™	4
Sports bar (i.e. Power Bar™)	1 average
Sugar	2 tbsp
Beverages and liquid supplements	
Soft drink/cordial	500 ml
Fruit juice	600 ml
Glucose powder/Glucodin™	2.5 tbsp
Sustagen™	4 tbsp
Polycose™/Maximum™	2.5 tbsp
Sustagen with milk	2 tbsp & 300 ml milk
Ensure Plus™	1 can
Sustagen tetrapak™	1.5
Sports drinks (e.g. Isosport™, Gatorade™, Exceed™)	750–800 ml
Ensure Powder™ (lactose-free)	80 g
Meal replacement fluid (Exceed Sport Meal Plus™, Gatorpro™)	1 can/tetrapak

In order to meet carbohydrate needs, frequent, small meals centred around nutritious carbohydrate foods should be eaten throughout the day. Examples include sandwiches and fruit. If children have difficulty in eating a high volume of relatively bulky foods (such as sandwiches, cereals, pasta, potatoes, etc.), sugars such as those found in sweet spreads (such as jam and honey) and sweetened drinks (such as cordials, soft drinks, fruit juices and sports drinks) can help ensure that sufficient carbohydrate is consumed. However, these latter foods should ideally be kept to less than 10 per cent of the total daily energy intake. Too much refined carbohydrates and sugars can lead to vitamin, mineral and fibre deficiencies, as well as a reduction in protein intake. Moreover, some high-sugar foods are also high in fat (for example, chocolate, pastries and rich desserts), and fat intake exceeding 30 per cent of the total daily energy should be avoided.

Prevention of glycogen depletion during training and competition depends upon regular and high carbohydrate intake.

Simple or complex carbohydrates?

Until recently, carbohydrates were considered to be either 'simple' or 'complex'. We generally assumed that simple carbohydrates were those released most quickly into the bloodstream, causing a rapid rise in blood sugar levels, while complex carbohydrates were digested more slowly and resulted in lower blood sugar levels. However, the speed at which carbohydrates influence blood sugar levels is now best explained by a term called the glycaemic index (GI).

Carbohydrates that have a relatively high GI are released quickly into the bloodstream after being eaten, while carbohydrates with a relatively low GI are released more slowly. As you can see from Table 13, some sweet foods such as those containing fructose (fruit sugar) have a low GI. The significance of a food's GI relates to the timing of a meal; if rapid energy (that is, glucose) needs to be made available to the muscles, then the athlete should eat foods with a high GI. This will be important if they are competing in a tournament and there is only an hour or so between matches or competition rounds. However, in some situations, rapid energy may not be necessary and a slower, more consistent energy 'release' may be suitable (for example, overnight). Low GI foods would then be more suitable.

Table 13 High and low glycaemic index foods

High GI foods:

Rice Bubbles™ and Cornflakes™

Puffed Wheat™ and Weet-bix™

Wholemeal and white bread

Puffed crispbread and water crackers

Calrose and sunbrown quick rice

Glucose

Bananas and watermelon

Low GI foods:

Porridge

Sultana Bran™

Long grain white rice

Instant noodles

Pasta

Fruit loaf

Mixed grain bread

Lentils

Kidney beans and baked beans

Apples

Milk and yoghurt

Fructose (fruit sugar)

Source: Adapted from *Nutrition Issues and Abstracts*, 'Glycaemic Index—An update and overview', No. 6, June 1995.

Increasing muscle glycogen levels

The traditional method for increasing muscle glycogen stores before exercise is termed carbohydrate loading and involves first deliberately depleting muscle glycogen stores (normally through exhaustive exercise), then eating a low-carbohydrate diet for three days before finally boosting muscle glycogen stores using a very high carbohydrate diet for four days. Although the procedure has been modified over the years, it is still used by some adults in preparation for endurance events. However, there is a modified approach which typically involves the athletes increasing their carbohydrate intake in the few days before competition, while at the same time reducing the training load (which is referred to as tapering). Teenagers will find this effective even though they may not exercise at the intensities and for the durations of exercise which are commonly associated with glycogen depletion. Nonetheless, there will be occasions (such as during a tournament, or when competing on consecutive days) when glycogen stores may be at risk of depletion. Carbohydrate intake in the days prior to and during such activities should therefore be increased, and there should be a decrease in training activity during the few days prior to such events in order to increase glycogen stores.

Protein

Due to body growth, the protein requirements for children and adolescents are higher than for adults. Having said that, however, the need for additional protein should be met by an increased total energy intake. That is, simply by eating more food, extra protein will be made available to the body and, because of this, protein supplements commonly available from health-food shops and gyms are not necessary. Protein intake for children and adolescents should range between 1.2 and 2 grams for every kilogram of their body weight (which equates to between 12 and 15 per cent of the total energy intake). Table 14 shows foods which provide 10 grams of protein.

Table 14 10-gram serves of protein

- 50 g of grilled fish
- 30 g of lean lamb or beef (cooked weight)
- 35 g of skinless chicken
- 300 ml of skimmed milk

- 70 g of cottage cheese
- 2 slices of reduced fat cheese
- 50 g of nuts
- 90 g of breakfast cereal
- 400 ml of soy milk
- 100 g of wholemeal bread
- 120 g of tofu

In rare circumstances when the diet fails to provide sufficient protein, an athlete may become more susceptible to fatigue, may be unable to build and maintain muscle mass, and may be slow to recover following injury. Attention should then be paid to increasing dietary protein intake.

An effective way to meet daily protein demands is to spread protein intake over five small meals per day, with approximately 35 grams of protein in any one meal or snack (see Table 14). Foods relatively high in protein are often accompanied by essential nutrients such as calcium, iron and zinc. Animal sources of protein include meat, poultry, fish and seafood, eggs and dairy products; these provide the best quality and balance of amino acids, which are the building blocks of muscle and many other structures in the body. Plant sources of protein include breads, breakfast cereals, rice, pasta, legumes and pulses, and commercially prepared vegetarian meat alternatives (for example. Nutmeat™ and Rediburger™). Foods derived from plants tend to be incomplete sources of the essential amino acids and are best combined with meat or fish. Nonetheless, a vegetarian diet can be entirely adequate in protein, provided it is carefully planned, balanced and includes a variety of protein sources.

Fats

Adults and children generally consume too much fat. The general consensus now is that cardiovascular disease begins in childhood, so fat intake in youngsters has long-term health implications. Nonetheless, some fats are essential to maintaining key functions, such as the health of blood vessels and production of some hormones, so complete avoidance of fats or a very low intake can be just as dangerous as an excessive intake.

Although fat is an important energy source during exercise, fatigue is not related to fat availability. In other words, we still have enough fat even when fatigued. Thus, 'fat loading' and consuming a high-fat diet before competition is not recommended for young athletes. The aim should be to eat a balanced, high-carbohydrate diet.

Vitamins and minerals

Small amounts of vitamins and minerals are needed to maintain health; they help produce energy, assist in the manufacture of red blood cells and are essential for tissue repair. Vitamin and mineral deficiencies result in early fatigue, increase susceptibility to illness and infections, and have been associated with slow recovery from wounds and injury. Importantly, if a person is eating a balanced diet (which can be assumed to provide all the necessary vitamins and minerals), vitamin and/or mineral supplementation will not enhance performance.

Vitamin deficiencies are rare. Nonetheless, they can result from poor dietary choices, food restriction and/or a biochemical deficiency. To ensure that adequate vitamins and mineral needs are met, it is best and most economical to improve the diet rather than resort to supplements. Thus, as more food is consumed, additional vitamins and minerals will inevitably be eaten. Table 15 lists the major food sources of various vitamins and minerals.

Table 15 Major vitamin and mineral sources

Vitamin A: Yellow and orange fruit and vegetables, eggs, dairy products, margarine and oils.

B Vitamins: Wholegrain bread and cereals, brown rice and pastas, Vegemite™, lean meats, dairy products, green leafy vegetables.

Vitamin C: Citrus, tropical and berry fruits, red capsicum and tomatoes.

Vitamin E: Wholegrain bread and cereals, wheatgerm, nuts and seeds, unsaturated oils.

Iron: Organ meats (e.g. liver), beef and other meats, turkey, chicken, fish and seafood. To a lesser extent, iron is found in eggs, green leafy vegetables, iron-enriched breads and cereals, dried fruits and legumes. (To increase iron absorption, include a source of vitamin C when eating lean red meat.)

Calcium: Dairy products and fortified soy milks (e.g. So Good™ and Good Life™). Lesser sources include fish, dark green vegetables, nuts and seeds, and wholegrains. (Adults should have 500 ml of milk and 200 g of yoghurt or 1 slice cheese per day, while children and adolescents need 750 ml of milk and 200 g of yoghurt or 1 slice of cheese.)

Calcium

Because calcium is important for the growth of bones, children need up to four servings of calcium-rich foods daily. The best sources of calcium are dairy products such as milk, cheese, yoghurt, etc. The lactose found in dairy products aids in calcium absorption. If children are allergic to milk products, then fortified soy milk alternatives (such as So Good™ and Good Life™) can be good sources of calcium; calcium supplements can also be taken.

Poor calcium intake during the growing years has been associated with a higher incidence of stress fractures in late adolescence and osteoporosis later in life. Although all the causes and consequences of osteoporosis are yet to be fully understood, there is no doubt that both young girls and boys need to maximise their calcium intake to promote maximal increases in bone density. Problems arise when young athletes reduce their energy intake while still maintaining a demanding exercise program; this results in a net loss of calcium and reduced bone density.

Iron

Iron is a mineral that is necessary for the production of haemoglobin; haemoglobin is needed to carry oxygen in the blood. Low iron intake can result in anaemia, which is associated with reduced exercise capacity, cramps, and decreased resistance to infection.

Iron deficiency is most common in females (due to their increased iron loss through menstruation) and in vegetarians. Other athletes who may be at risk of iron depletion include those who have frequent nosebleeds and those that have had an illness or taken medication resulting in blood loss. Excessive high-impact exercise may also lead to iron deficiency, as will consuming poorly balanced diets and diets low in energy. Athletes at risk of iron deficiency should have regular blood tests performed by a sports physician to check their haemoglobin and ferritin (iron storage) levels. In some cases, iron supplementation may be recommended.

In order to meet their iron needs, children should be encouraged to consume red meats, poultry, fish and other seafood. Foods such as legumes (kidney beans, lentils), eggs, wholegrain and fortified cereals (Weet-bix™, Vitabrits™, Sustain™, Special K™), and dark green vegetables (spinach, broccoli) also provide some iron, though when compared to red meat, iron from these foods will be less easily absorbed by the body.

TRAINING AND COMPETITION DIETS

Before training or competition

The training diet has to meet fuel and nutrient needs during periods of high energy output, establish healthy long-term eating habits, maintain an appropriate fat-to-muscle ratio, and promote rapid recovery from exercise.

The key nutritional priorities for maximising performance in both training and competition are maximising muscle and liver glycogen stores and maintaining adequate fluid levels.

If a balanced, high-carbohydrate diet has been consumed in the days immediately preceding competition, then the muscles' glycogen stores should be relatively high. A large meal comprised of easily digestible sources of carbohydrate should be consumed three to four hours before exercise, while a carbohydrate snack should be consumed at regular intervals right up to the start of competition. The current view is that a high glycaemic carbohydrate food (such as sports drinks or confectionery) consumed up to ten minutes prior to exercise may benefit performance.

Timing and meal selection prior to exercise will depend on individual preference and appetite, as well as when the event is due to begin. Fat (for example, cheese) and fibre (such as high-fibre cereals) should be avoided close to competition so as to minimise stomach and gut discomfort and promote rapid absorption of the carbohydrates. Most importantly, the meal should consist of familiar foods which the athlete feels comfortable eating. Adequate fluid intake is also essential. If an athlete is too nervous to eat, he or she may prefer a liquid meal such as Gatorpro™, Sustagen™, Exceed Sport Meal Plus™, Ensure™ or a low-fat milk drink (such as a banana smoothie made with skimmed milk and honey). Examples of suitable pre-competition meals include:

- pancakes, cereals, bread, toast and fruit;
- pasta with a tomato-based sauce; or
- sports drinks, cordials, soft drinks and fresh fruit smoothies.

During exercise

Many children compete in tournaments and intermittent activities that last a number of hours. It is therefore desirable to consume carbohydrates and fluids during the course of such events. It should be possible to experiment with both liquid sources (sports drinks, diluted cordials and glucose syrups), and food sources of carbohydrate (such as sports bars, bananas, sandwiches, etc.) in training, to determine combinations which are most acceptable and effective at maintaining energy levels.

Post-exercise

Children should be encouraged to eat approximately 1 gram of carbohydrate per kilogram of their body weight in the first 30 minutes after exercise, and to continue this intake every two hours until the usual daily intake of carbohydrate is reached. Table 16 provides a list of 50-gram serves of carbohydrate drinks and snacks that are ideal for post-exercise recovery.

The fastest rate of recovery following exercise is achieved by consuming food and drinks with a moderate to high glycaemic index (see Table 13). Examples of these are sports drinks, glucose confectionery, cordials and soft drinks (non-caffeine), fruits such as watermelon and bananas, as well as bread, potatoes and some wheat-based breakfast cereals. Fruit provides fructose, which can help to replace liver glycogen stores.

FLUID REPLACEMENT

Water is essential for the process of sweating, which in turn is critical for maintaining body temperature within safe limits

Table 16 50-gram serves of carbohydrate drinks and snacks

- 750 ml sports drink (e.g. Isosport™, Gatorade™, Exceed Fluid and Energy Replacement™, Powerade™, Sport Plus™)
- 750 ml cordial, 500 ml juice or non-cola soft drink
- 250–400 ml Sustagen™, Ensure™, Exceed Sport Meal™, or reduced fat milkshake/smoothie
- 1 serve of Gatorpro™ or Exceed Sport Meal Plus™
- 200–250 ml 'carbo-loader' drink (e.g. Gatorlode™ or Exceed High Carbohydrate Source™)
- 50 g jelly beans or jelly lollies
- 1 round of thick jam/honey/banana sandwiches
- 3 pieces of fruit
- 2–3 muesli bars
- 1 sports bar (e.g. Power Bar™, Exceed Sport Bar™)
- bowl of cereal with reduced fat milk and banana
- bowl of fruit salad and tub of fruit yoghurt
- 2 large pancakes with lots of syrup
- bowl of pasta/rice with low-fat toppings

Note that most 'fast foods' are low in carbohydrates.

and preventing heat illness. Failure to lose excess heat from the body will impair performance and can be potentially fatal.

Children, compared with adults, have a higher surface area to volume ratio and this favours heat gain from the sun. Coupled with this, children sweat less and tend to have a lower capacity to lose heat. To compound these differences, children generally do not drink enough; it is worth remembering that thirst is a poor indicator of fluid needs. Children must therefore be reminded to drink at regular, frequent intervals, and parents and coaches should ensure that children have easy access to fluid during training and competition.

For every kilogram of body weight lost during exercise, a litre of water (preferably water which is mildly sugared (5 per cent) and salted (0.5–1 per cent)) needs to be consumed. The dissolved sugar helps to replace energy lost during exercise, while the salt assists in the uptake and retention of the water. There is no need to add anything other than sugar and salt to water for fluid and partial energy replacement.

Fluid replacement should begin immediately following exercise and should continue until normal body weight is regained. Possible drinks to use for fluid replacement include water, sports drinks (for example, Isosport™, Gatorade™ or Exceed™), carbohydrate loading drinks (Gatorlode™ or Exceed Hi-carb™), cordials, non-cola soft drinks, and meal replacement/milk drinks (Sustagen™, Exceed Sport Meal™ or a low-fat milk smoothie). Cool drinks are more refreshing and palatable than warm ones. Practical tips for fluid and electrolyte replacement include:

- Hydration before exercise (that is, consuming regular drinks all day and up to/during the hour prior to training or competition).
- Ensuring that urine is clear and dilute before exercise.
- Replacement of fluid is increased when a large volume is consumed. Thus, rather than small sips, children should be encouraged to take in as much fluid as they can comfortably tolerate.
- Weighing before and after exercise and replacing approximately 1 litre of fluid for every 1 kilogram of weight lost.
- Consume cool fluids.

Drinks containing approximately 5 per cent carbohydrate (for example, 50 grams of glucose or glucose polymers dissolved in 1 litre of water) and low levels of salt (0.5–1 per cent) can help to replace fluids and carbohydrates lost during exercise. The choice made by an individual athlete or team may depend on taste preference, cost and availability. The most important ingredients in a sports drink are water, carbohydrate (preferably glucose) and sodium (found in table salt). Additional ingredients are only important for improving the taste of a drink.

Deliberate weight (that is, water) loss in the lead-up to competition is an extremely dangerous practice and must be avoided. Quite aside from the inevitable cost to performance, there is an increased risk of dehydration and heat illness.

ERGOGENIC AIDS

We had initially intended to include a large section reviewing ergogenic aids (such as creatine, carnitine, sodium bicarbonate, etc.). However, since the health risks of such compounds are unknown for pre-adolescents, our advice is that sensible dietary strategies alone are adequate to meet the demands of both growth and activity.

WEIGHT CONTROL

Weight control is a socially contentious and sensitive issue. Problems associated with perceptions of body image include bulimia (binge eating and vomiting) and anorexia nervosa (both of which are dealt with in more detail below). The term 'overweight' is misleading; 'over-fat' is usually the more accurate term, in which case, there are sensible strategies which can achieve and maintain realistic goals. However, there should be careful assessment of any health risk before any modification in eating behaviour is made. An issue that complicates matters is when children compete in sports and activities such as ballet, skating, diving and gymnastics, where leanness and appearance during performance are important.

Gains in body fat often result from consuming too much fat and not enough carbohydrate in the diet; eating too much, particularly late in the day; skipping meals, especially breakfast and lunch; and bingeing between meals and/or late at night, also contribute to fat gains. In addition, energy expenditure (that is, exercise) may be too low for the volume of calories being consumed.

With fat loss, there should be no more than a 0.5–1 kilogram reduction in body weight per week. Any more than this will translate into loss of muscle, and performance will worsen. In addition, it is sensible to spread food intake over five or six small meals per day, rather than two or three larger meals; a balanced intake of nutrients must still be maintained. It may also be necessary to change poor eating habits, such as eating when bored, stressed or depressed. Parallel to modifying energy intake, low-intensity, long-duration exercise (such as walking or cycling) is best for promoting fat loss while maintaining muscle tissue.

Eating disorders

Anorexia and bulimia often develop in adolescence, with girls being more prone to these problems than boys. Girls tend to have a greater preoccupation with dieting, which is associated with peer pressure and sociocultural influences. Coupled with this, the make-up of an elite athlete is associated with perfectionism and conformation.

According to the American Psychiatric Association, anorexia nervosa is characterised by the following:

- refusal to maintain body weight over a minimal normal weight for age and height;
- intense fear of gaining weight or becoming fat, even when underweight;
- disturbance in the way in which one's body weight, size or shape is experienced (for example, the person feels 'fat' even when he or she is thin);
- in girls, absence of at least three consecutive menstrual cycles when they are otherwise expected to occur.

Bulimia nervosa is characterised by the following:

- recurrent episodes of binge eating (rapid consumption of a large amount of food in a discrete period of time);
- a feeling of lack of control over eating behaviour during the eating binges;
- the person regularly engages in self-inflicted vomiting, use of laxatives or diuretics, strict dieting or fasting, or vigorous exercise in order to prevent weight gain;
- a minimum average of two binge eating episodes a week for at least three months;
- persistent overconcern with body shape and weight.

As Stanton (1994) points out, many athletes may not quite meet these criteria, yet still have underlying eating problems. Careful attention to peculiar eating habits and obsessive behaviour may prevent a worsening of the problem.

There is an increased risk of amenorrhoea (that is, loss of periods) in girls and women with eating disorders, and this is associated with reduced bone mineral density and an increased risk of stress fractures. In addition, gastrointestinal problems, anxiety and depression, impaired performance, longer recovery time following exercise and an increased risk of injury occur in athletes who have eating disorders.

Treatment involves early counselling by health professionals (dietitians or counsellors), parents and coaches. If the cause of the problem can be identified, nutritional counselling, psychotherapy, family therapy, pharmacological therapy and possibly medical intervention may be needed. Parents play a vital role in ensuring that the nutritional needs of children are met.

Bulking-up, anabolic steroids and growth hormone

As explained in Chapter 5, children and pre-adolescents have a limited capacity to significantly increase the size of their muscles, even when they perform resistance training. This is because levels of the male hormone testosterone remain relatively low up to puberty.

There is evidence that an increasing number of adolescents are taking anabolic steroids in an attempt to increase muscle mass (for appearance and to enhance sports performance). Anabolic steroids are chemicals manufactured to mimic the actions of testosterone, and they promote the growth and development of many body tissues, including muscle, bone, skin, hair and sex organs. Quite aside from the ethical concerns, anabolic steroid abuse may interrupt growth in children, contribute to liver disease, increase the risk of heart disease and cause psychological disturbances. Use of anabolic steroids must be strongly discouraged.

Clues to detecting whether someone may be taking anabolic steroids include abrupt changes in their behaviour, an increased incidence of nosebleeds and acne, abnormal increases in their size and strength, and abnormally low levels of HDL (high-density lipoproteins) cholesterol in the blood.

Growth hormone is not an anabolic steroid but is a chemical messenger that plays a central role in promoting growth from birth. It is secreted naturally by the pituitary gland. Some athletes therefore take growth hormone in an attempt to increase their size and improve performance. If growth hormone is given to children, the risks include gigantism, enlarged but weakened muscles, cardiovascular disease and diabetes.

The message is clear: do not rely on artificial means to improve performance. Instead, combine sound nutritional practices with sensible training.

In conclusion, nutrition plays a central role in both training and performance. There is no doubt that the fittest athlete or player can lose an event or game as a result of poor nutritional preparation or inadequate recovery from a previous exercise session. Clearly, failure to recognise the importance of dietary practices in the overall scheme of performance will prevent an athlete from reaching his or her full potential. From the health perspective, sensible eating habits developed in childhood are vital for reducing the risks of developing heart disease, diabetes, high blood pressure and obesity later in life.

SUMMARY

✓ Energy intake must be sufficient to meet growth needs and the additional demands of activity (training and performance). Healthy snacks throughout the day can help to meet energy demands and avoid shortfalls in calorie intake.

✓ Between 55 and 60 per cent of the total energy consumed each day should be in the form of carbohydrate. Carbohydrate is stored in the liver and muscles as glycogen, which is the most important source of energy for 90 per cent of activities. Inadequate intake of carbohydrate will result in early fatigue during exercise, lethargy and poor concentration.

✓ Foods with a high glycaemic index should be consumed as soon as possible following exercise. These will promote rapid replenishment of glycogen stores and a faster recovery.

✓ Carbohydrate intake needs to be increased in the two or three days before a tournament or competition. This should parallel a decrease in the amount of exercise performed during the same period.

✓ Fat should be kept to less than 30 per cent of the total energy intake. Fatigue is not associated with low fat levels and, because of this, fat loading before competition should be avoided.

✓ A normal, balanced diet will provide enough protein to meet the body's needs, provided enough calories are being consumed. Protein supplements are only necessary in exceptional circumstances.

✓ Calcium and iron are important for bone health and blood function, respectively. Children and adolescents must ensure that their diets provide adequate amounts of these minerals.

✓ Carbohydrate and fluid are critical nutrients for exercise performance. Fluid replacement can be enhanced when a small amount of salt is added to water; similarly, sugar in water can help delay fatigue if consumed during exercise and will enhance recovery if consumed immediately following exercise.

✓ Fat loss is best achieved by moderating fat intake, eating regularly and undertaking low-intensity, long-duration exercise.

✓ Anabolic steroids and growth hormone have extremely serious side-effects and should be avoided at all costs.

Sensible eating, coupled with a carefully designed training program, will improve performance legally and with minimal risks to health.

Further reading

Chapter 1: Changes to the body during childhood

Blimkie, C.J.R. 1989 'Age- and sex-associated variation in strength during childhood' *Perspectives in Exercise Science and Sports Medicine* eds C. Gisolfi and D. Lamb, Benchmark Press, Indianapolis, IN.

Goldberg, B. 1995 *Sports and Exercise for Children with Chronic Health Conditions*, Human Kinetics, Champaign, IL.

Lohman, T.G. 1986 'Applicability of body composition techniques and constants for children and youth' *Exercise and Sport Sciences Reviews* ed. K.B. Pandolf, Macmillan, New York, pp. 325–57.

Malina, R.M. 1989 'Growth and maturation: normal variation and effect of training' *Perspectives in Exercise Science and Sports Medicine* eds C. Gisolfi and D. Lamb, Benchmark Press, Indianapolis, IN.

Pate, R.R. and Shepherd, R.J. 1989 'Characteristics of physical fitness in youth' *Perspectives in Exercise Science and Sports*

Medicine eds C. Gisolfi and D. Lamb, Benchmark Press, Indianapolis, IN.

Reaburn, P. and Jenkins, D. (eds) 1996 *Training for Speed and Endurance*, Allen & Unwin, Sydney.

Rowland, T.W. 1996 *Developmental Exercise Physiology*, Human Kinetics, Champaign, IL.

Sports Medicine Australia 1997 *Safety Guidelines for Children in Sport and Recreation*, Sports Medicine Australia, Canberra. Available from: Sports Medicine Australia, PO Box 897, Belconnen, ACT 2616.

Wilmore, J. and Costill, D. 1999 *Physiology of Sport and Exercise*, Human Kinetics, Champaign, IL.

Chapter 2: Chronic health disorders and exercise

Goldberg, B. (ed.) 1995 *Sports and Exercise for Children with Chronic Health Conditions*, Human Kinetics, Champaign, IL.

Micheli, L.J. (ed.) 1995 *Clinics in Sports Medicine: The Young Athlete*, W.B. Saunders, Philadelphia, PA.

Chapter 3: Management of common injuries

Hochsculer, S.H. (ed.) 1990 *The Spine in Sports*, Hanley and Belfus, Philadelphia.

Micheli, L.J. (ed.) 1995 *Clinics in Sports Medicine: The Young Athlete*, W.B. Saunders, Philadelphia, PA.

Reid, D.C. (ed.) 1992 *Sports Injury Assessment and Rehabilitation*, Churchill Livingstone, New York.

Chapter 4: Training for speed, endurance and flexibility

Alter, S. 1996 *Science of Flexibility*, 2nd edn, Human Kinetics, Champaign, IL.

Alter, S. 1998 *Sport Stretch*, Human Kinetics, Champaign, IL.

Dintiman, G. and Ward, R. 1988 *Sport Speed*, Leisure Press, Champaign, IL.

Ellison, D. 1999 *Performance Stretching*, Human Kinetics, Champaign, IL.

Newsholme, E., Leech, T. and Duester, G. 1994 *Keep on Running*, John Wiley & Sons, Chichester, UK.

Reaburn, P. and Jenkins, D. 1996 *Training for Speed and Endurance*, Allen & Unwin, Sydney.

Rowland, T.W. 1996 *Developmental Exercise Physiology*, Human Kinetics, Champaign, IL.

Chapter 5: Training for strength

Baechle, T.R. (ed.) 1994 *Essentials of Strength and Conditioning*, Human Kinetics, Champaign, IL.

Baechle, T.R. and Groves, B.R. 1992 *Weight Training: Steps to Success*, Human Kinetics, Champaign, IL.

Chapter 6: Enhancing recovery

Calder, A. 1996 'Recovery training' *Training for Speed and Endurance* (eds) P. Reaburn and D. Jenkins, Allen & Unwin, Sydney.

Calder, A. 1992 *Recovery Planner*, available from the Australian Coaching Council. PO Box 176, Belconnen ACT 2616 (a useful planning tool for recovery training).

Chapter 7: Nutrition and exercise

Burke, L. 1992 *The Complete Guide to Food for Sports Performance*, Allen & Unwin, Sydney.

Burke, L. and Deakin, V. (eds) 1994 *Clinical Sports Nutrition*, McGraw-Hill, Sydney.

Grundy, M. 1994 'Foods children use for sports performance' *Sport Health* vol. 12, no. 2, p. 41.

Stanton, R. 1994 *Eating for Peak Performance*, 2nd edn, Allen & Unwin, Sydney.

Williams, M.H. 1995 *Nutrition for Fitness and Sport*, 4th edn, WCB McGraw-Hill, Sydney.

Index

PEAK PERFORMANCE

Training and nutritional strategies for sport

JOHN HAWLEY and LOUISE BURKE
Foreword by Tim Noakes

Whether your aim is to win an Olympic medal, to reach the finals in a national competition or just to finish an endurance event with a smile on your face, there is a common goal. All athletes strive to achieve their best on the day of competition. Your tools are effective training techniques and a great nutrition program.

Peak Performance is a one-stop text for coaches, athletes and students of sports science who want to improve their knowledge and sporting performance by the application of scientific training and nutritional principles. It combines the results of state of the art research, from the world leaders in these fields, together with practical guidelines to meet the challenges of daily training and nutrition in the preparation for competition. It investigates:

- the body's power systems and how the body responds to training
- how to measure performance and test fitness specific to the needs of your sport
- devising particular training programs for endurance, team or power sports
- special strategies to help you get it right on the day
- clever eating before, during and after a session—either training or competition—to ensure your best possible performance
- eating to maximise recovery between training sessions
- which supplements are best and how to use them
- appraisal of the latest scientific aids and strategies (heart-rate monitors, altitude and hill training, warming up and warming down, drafting and pacing)
- the limits to athletic performance.

SPORT/FITNESS

1 86448 469 1

TRAINING FOR SPEED AND ENDURANCE

Edited by PETER REABURN and DAVID JENKINS

Training for sport has developed at a bewildering pace during the 1990s and has left coaches and athletes struggling to keep up with all the theories on offer and then to apply the most effective ones to their daily training regimens.

The contributors to *Training for Speed and Endurance* are sports specialists keen to bridge the gap between laboratory findings and athlete preparation. They are all involved in the training and preparation of elite athletes and their aim in writing this book has been to provide practical guidelines for developing and maintaining speed and endurance fitness for both individuals and team players.

Areas covered include:

- exercise physiology essentials
- speed training methods
- endurance training methods
- periodisation of speed and endurance
- conditioning the team player
- recovery training
- nutrition for sports performance
- injury treatment and prevention

Training for Speed and Endurance will make sense of all the new techniques and latest research. It will be of interest to anyone wishing to gain up-to-date information on training principles and will be of particular value to those individuals or team players who need to focus on speed and endurance. The book is an excellent resource for coaches, individual athletes, health and physical educators of senior students and tertiary students of sports science.

Peter Reaburn and **David Jenkins** are former representative Rugby Union players who both now lecture in exercise physiology.

SPORT/FITNESS

1 86448 120 X

GOOD SKIN

Safe and simple skin care for today's world

HUGH MOLLOY and GARRY EGGER
Foreword by Dr Norman Swan

' . . . There is much wisdom in this book, and the remedies are simple.'
Terence J. Ryan, Emeritus Professor of Dermatology, Oxford

This is a book about your body's largest organ—your skin. More specifically, it's a book about modern skin problems and their possible causes and management.

Do you or your family suffer with

- dry, rough or scaly skin?
- unexplained morning sneezing and a runny nose?
- persistent acne?
- limp, lifeless, stringy or greasy hair?
- dark rings around the eyes?
- recurrent tinea?
- disturbed sleep?

All these problems are closely related to our modern environment—we spend a lot of time in excessively dry air, are often overheated and are obsessed with cleanliness. These three factors are responsible for conditions ranging from persistent acne to eczema and psoriasis. *Good Skin* explains why and provides simple, safe, non-invasive and inexpensive solutions.

Dr Hugh Molloy has been a visiting skin specialist at a number of teaching hospitals in New South Wales. He is in practice in Sydney and is currently an Emeritus Consultant to the Department of Dermatology at the Royal Prince Alfred Hospital, Sydney. **Dr Garry Egger** is Director of the Centre for Health Promotion and Research in Sydney and an Adjunct Professor of Health Sciences at Deakin University.

HEALTH

1 86508 092 6